NATURE And PURPOSE Of DISEASE:

Definitive Guide for Peoples with Melanin

by

Henry L. N. Anderson, Ed.D.,

Author of *Helping Hand: 8-Day Diet Programs*

with

T.C. Fry, D.Sc.,

Author of *The Great AIDS Hoax*

INTRODUCTION by
VIVIAN VIRGINIA VETRANO, DC, MD

First Edition Printing, August 2001
Revised Second Printing, September 2002

ISBN#: 1-564-11263-2

Published by American University Publishers
P.O. Box 4277
Inglewood, CA 90309-4277
(A division of City University Los Angeles)

Printed in the U. S. A.
by
CONQUERING BOOKS, L.L.C.
210 East Arrowhead Drive #1
Charlotte, N. C. 28213
(704) 509-2226 - publish@conqueringbooks.com

Knowledge is the greatest of our benighted and purblind world. Knowledge of how to live; knowledge of ***the nature and purpose of disease****; knowledge of the evils and futility of treatment; knowledge of the truth about life--this is the need of the whole world today.*

- T. C. Fry, 1974

Table of Contents

Acknowledgments

Had my late wife, Agnes Alberta Fox Anderson (February 1935- May 1997) objected to my traveling alone to Carnival in Rio de Janeiro, Brazil I would not have sat next to Kenneth Desrosiers, who sometime later became a Natural Hygienist, and introduced me to one of its chief spokespersons, T. C. Fry. Had "Mr. Fry" not taken time with me, and showed patience, tolerance and an appreciation of my doubts and questions, I might not have changed by own lifestyle to that recommended by the research and promulgation of Dr. Herbert M. Shelton, and others.

Had I not learned from "my teachers" and demonstrated in my own life the practical benefits of pursuing a "healthful living," plant-based lifestyle, I would not have had the courage or the information to be supportive to Agnes when, in 1993, she was diagnosed with "metastasized cancer in the lungs and beyond" (and was given "about three months" to live!).

Given the choice of following the path of conventional medicine or what I had come to advocate as a more natural, more redemptive, and more optimistic approach to responding to disease symptoms, Agnes made the choice to follow in the path of Natural Hygiene.

I applaud her to this very day; and because of her courage I was re-inspired to see relationships: between early life exposures to toxic substances and later symptoms of disease; between dietary patterns and internal bodily structures; between emotional reservoir and mental garbage; between lifestyle 'causes' and disease symptom 'effects.'

This book was begun during the four years Agnes and I renewed our living according to our new hygienic beliefs—long beyond the predicted time of her demise!

She encouraged its exploration of truth, and its passion to share whatever wisdom it could reasonably verify. T. C. Fry spoke to Agnes on the telephone at my request; he 'encouraged' her to forego traditional medical treatments, especially chemotherapy and he wrote portions for this volume. Then, without warming or anticipation, T. C. Fry was suddenly no more. That was September 6, 1996; Agnes died May 14, 1997.

From 1997 to 2001, this volume has been a work in progress. Thanks to the caring support of Dr. Margie Nell Johnson, my new wife, who insisted that I persevere, and Dr. Vivian Virginia Vetrano who "explained" T. C. Fry to the rest of us and has written the **Introduction** for this volume.

There were others—Tarik Ricard, Harvey Diamond, James Michael Lennon, Dr. and Mrs. Charles Jay Young, my three grown children and their companions and eight grand-children, in addition to friends (living and now dead), siblings and family —whom I acknowledge, and I am indebted to for what appears in this volume.

I am also grateful to all those involved in the publishing of this volume, just as I am to those who dare to read and consider its implications.

—Henry L. N. Anderson

Dedication

To Empress Verdiacee "Tiari" Washitaw-Turner Goston, Author of *Return of the Ancient Ones*, and reigning Empress of Empire Washitaw de Dugdahmoundyah (Exodus 20:20-26), "The Oldest Indigenous People on Earth" (U.N. Designation #215-93). And to Reatter Ashford Lonon, my maternal grandmother (who so resembled Her Emperial Highness, but for time and distance they could have been blood sisters)!

Introduction

By V. V. Vetrano, D.C., hM.D., M.D.

Reading this book may scare you, astound you, shock you, give you hope, inform you of things few people know, or just entertain you, but you can be sure that if you understand and use its concepts, it will change your life forever, for the better. If you fear learning something new, or if you fear knowing something that very few people know, or if you fear following a different path than your family or friends, then put this book down now. But, if you want to be in possession of knowledge that can save your life, make you healthier, happier, and which will help elevate you and all the peoples of the world then read on, my friend.

Like many people, when first reading about Natural Hygiene and learning the principles of life, it is almost like getting a shock treatment. You are left stunned. Then because of what you have learned, you need to put a vacuum cleaner to your brain and suck out all the propaganda that has been stuffed into your mind about health and disease since you were born. Only after extracting all the disinformation, can you insert new laws, ideas and principles that propel you into a way of life that is totally different from the one you now lead. When you follow Nature's Laws as taught by Natural Hygienists you are promised happiness, freedom from pain, sickness, and chronic degenerative disease, instead of the misery, sickness, starvation and death that come from living indifferently to your body's needs. You may be able to pull yourself out of the dumps of poverty from improved mental clarity. Finally when it is time to die it will not be after years of suffering, but easy, just like a flower fading away. You will decide you have lived long enough, just as the Amerindians did, and just pass on without having to suffer from all the drugs, surgery, mutilation, injections, and intravenous feedings in the long run.

When I first read *Superior Nutrition* by Dr. Herbert M. Shelton, the author's ideas and laws struck me as logical and so truthful that I could not negate or argue any part of the book. I became a Hygienist overnight at the age of 18. I threw out all my bottles of vitamin and mineral supplements, brewers yeast and everything that had been jammed into my brain as promoters of health by those who wanted to commercialize on health. Then I went to the fruit and vegetable market and bought the real carriers of vitamins and minerals, the only sources that can really be used by the body. Only fresh unprocessed fruits, vegetables, and nuts supply us with our nutrients.

What fun I had eating meals out of those things that are commonly thought of as desserts or snacks. I ate meals of peaches, pears and apples and my taste buds reveled and thrilled to the natural sugars. I was ecstatic with the pleasure of dining on such delicious sweet meats. Every meal was and still is a banquet. While eating, the thought that came to my mind was: "I can eat all of these delicious foods and know that my body is not being robbed of its minerals like it would be if I ate that much sugar in the form of cakes, candy, pies and pastry."

The most wonderful thing about the Natural Diet is that as you continue on this path, you develop a lightness and vigor that you never thought possible. On heavy cooked foods, you feel lethargic and unable to think clearly. Cooked food pulls you down, but when you begin to eat live food—Wow! You can't believe the buoyancy and lightness and pep you have. It is almost like floating above the world on Harry Potter's "firebolt broom."

But, the marvelous thing about what you are going to learn in this book is not just about food and feeding, but it is about the very nature of your wonderful self. How you are self-healing, self-repairing, and self-regenerating. How you can determine your own health-fate. You will learn that you can be healthy simply by supplying the conditions of health. Rather than something you cannot see invading your body making you sick, you will find out that you can live in such a way that your own body easily destroys all so called “infectious” invaders.

More significant that that is the fact that you are master of your own body, can control and direct your life the way you desire, and produce health or disease at will! If you follow the Laws of Nature then the ultimate result will be genuine, beautiful, happy health. But by following the easy common way of living you will produce disease.

This book delves into Cause and Effect in a way that I have never yet read about. Even though it seems a little complicated at first, it is very logical and enlightening. It makes you want to read more about the spiritual part of yourself.

Young people who are now programmed to care so little for their precious physical bodies need to discover this book right now, before their brains, livers, kidneys, digestive systems and all their other vital organs have been damaged and partly destroyed by medications, hard drugs, and nutrition-less food, and also by all things that sap vitality and put them on the path of death well before their time.

By learning and using the principles set out in this book you will be able to preserve youth much longer than the average person with false life principles. You will learn to prize and respect the wonderful physical and mental body that God gave you to use in this world. Instead of treating it with disdain and thinking that you are invincible you will learn to take care of yourself. You are not invincible but you are a self-healing organism. You are hurting yourself when you waste your precious life away by partying every night and indulging in all the current follies that don’t bring real happiness. A questionable ephemeral short bit of artificial joy is not worth the damage it does to your body and mind, nor the future pain and suffering that is in store for you by unhealthful behavior. You will learn that true joy and true euphoria are brought about by the normal, natural things of life and not by drugs, alcohol and all the non-naturals that people take for granted that they should have to be happy. You will find out that: If you have to drink to be happy, you are not happy and never will be. If you take stimulants to get going, you are destroying your get going ability.

The teachings in this book should be put before every young person in the world. In it you will find the key to genuine happiness and health without drugs. Drugs and medications cause future misery just as they do to those athletes who ruin their lives by taking steroids. If you know and live by this method you won't devolve into disease but you will evolve into better and better health. Anyone really healthy is happy within. All the trillions of tiny cells in your body are joyously happy when nourished properly and when they are not bombarded with poisons.

Changing your life style is not an easy road to travel because you will be living a way that is different from most of the people around you. Another reason making the change is difficult, is that your nervous system has been conditioned. You are conditioned into eating and drinking all sorts of concoctions that are not good for you. Places like sitting in front of TV are the trigger that makes you automatically go to the refrigerator and encourages the munching syndrome. It takes a long time to undo the conditioning and you will need to cultivate patience and perseverance to succeed.

Are you willing to pay the price? Are you willing to be strong enough to dance to your own intelligent drumbeat? Are you willing to become what God wanted you to be? Are you willing to begin the self-discipline that will help you achieve a life of pleasure and abundance on your own and be one out of a million that knows the truth about health and disease? It is up to you. You are the master of your own soul and physical body. You don't have to remain in the dark slums and mud puddles. You can get out by using your God Given Intelligence. Learn to think on your own and do not follow the crowd. They are often ignorant and play follow the leader over the cliff.

This book is appropriate for the general public, but in order to attract those people with increased melanin, who need specific information to protect themselves from political infractions and conspiracy, a subtitle was placed on the cover. When speaking to Dr. Margie Anderson, the wife of the principal author, she explained the inclusion of the world melanin in the book's subtitle. I remarked that, "Everybody has melanin. Some people just have more of it." She chuckled and said, "That's a new way of looking at it."

People with more melanin do not usually come across many books like this and it was thought by the author that a subtitle about the people with more melanin would catch their eye and pique their curiosity. If it does, then Dr. Henry Anderson will have been instrumental in bringing enlightenment to all those people in the world whose skin contains more melanin in varying shades from light to dark.

There are so many good things in this book that to tell you about them all would give away the special thoughts in the book. So, read on young people. The rewards are phenomenal. Read on older people. It's never too late to stop poisoning yourself. The book makes you think about life, the laws of cause and effect and the effects of causes. You will puzzle, and think and think some more and come up with many new paradigms worth fighting for. Actually, when you think of it, the cause of disease is "life." If there were no life there would be no reason for disease. Whatever Great Power caused life, it is there, and since all life is more or less physical it has its special needs. If the needs are not met your life devolves and decays into chaos. It will remain in chaos until it returns itself to its natural state of health because that is what it was built to do.

—Vivian Virginia Vetrano, D.C., hM.D., M.D.
Barksdale, TX. June 28, 2001

Author's Preface

Writers are also humans, as much so if not more so than 'ordinary folks.' And, we feel and often live with our frustrations for long, unforgiving periods of time! Too often, we are at a loss when we consider sharing our innermost doubts, fears, and waning optimism.

I must tell you this: though I am ever so certain of the relative wisdom of these writings, and am ever so convinced the principles upon which they are based are life saving, life preserving and life improving, I fear so little heed will be taken, I question whether this writing justifies the time spent and the passion expended.

My problem is very personal—no doubt, too personal. It is the dichotomy of respecting everyone's 'free will,' given by The Creator, "Mother Nature," on the one hand, and on the other, knowing how we are all subject to the proposition that a healthy, long, happy and quality life is co-dependent on how one consumes (eats, drinks, exercises, rests, and believes) throughout all his or her years.

But, there are issues that are not considered in this volume. Often thought of, and treated as if they were "disease conditions," they are, more specifically, invasions or "attacks" or, perhaps, 'assaults' on our individual organisms. These 'attacks' or assaults are as 'harmless' as the "common cold," or they might be as fatal as "metastasized cancer!"

The first of these is the notion of *germs*. Some writers have said that the late billionaire, Howard Hughes, had such a fear of germs much of his environment was kept sterile! The world renown pop singer and entertainer, Michael Jackson, is said to once cut short a trip to Africa because he could not endure the smell of body odor and the thought of germs in the air, on people's hands, and possibly in the food and water.

But, germs are not only "not the enemy" or the deterrent to good health, they are, in fact, a necessary factor in optimum wellness. **The innate purpose accorded to germs is to return organic matter to Nature.** As **rust** transforms metal back to essential elements, germs ultimately assist in re-cycling natural or organic elements. So, like dedicated police officers, they are more friendly than hostile.

So long as the amount of rust is controlled, or the use of police power is tempered or the 'number' of germs appearing on one site is regulated, life maintains its normal flora. Excesses violate 'Natural Law' and there are consequences directly brought on by the excess—excesses from which no violator may 'escape' (wealth and power notwithstanding!).

Bacteria are 'germs' that specialize, if you will, in deterioration. They are the chief, active, agent in the decomposition of organic matter. Bacteria thrive when the conditions are favorable. An uncovered body sore will encourage the multiplication of bacteria, as will unclean moisture on the body, the carcass of a dead animal, or the fecal matter of humans (perhaps, potentially the most deadly of all!).

There is also a 'divine' kinship among bacteria, vultures, sharks, catfish, and even beasts of prey. Each plays a vital role in the Natural Order of Existence. They get rid of dead or wasting matter. They help keep species strong by hastening the departure of the dying and the dead.

Parasites, on the other hand, might be considered 'dangerous nuisances.' That is, they are not partial to man or to animal; they 'accept' either host, depending upon their species and location.

In some tropical areas, children and some adults are more "at risk" from 'blood sucking parasites,' 'free loaders,' and tape worms than from 'influenza,' so-called "childhood diseases" or vehicular and other accidents.

Water-borne parasites are to be found in our own local ponds, sometimes in public drinking water, and in such flesh as is used for food, i.e., shell and other fishes, and in certain animals, especially pork, chicken, and beef.

'Assaults' on the body which have as their primary source parasites, are often considered "infectious." It is commonly believed, for example, that a person who has "a cold" can and will "infect" those around—by touching, breathing or sharing, common air space. The fallacy of this notion of "contagion" is only reinforced when several people are "exposed" to the same "tinted" beef, milk, water, fish, or toxic air from high-rise air conditioning systems! In all such cases, "slight of hand" occurs: **what appears to be one thing is actually quite another.**

People who drink the same poison tend to show the same ill effects. Cholera, for example, was thought to be highly contagious and extremely deadly! Drinking water supplies were 'purified' and 'cholera' virtually disappeared.

Exposure to poisonous substances—whether antibiotics in animal products, pesticides in vegetables and fruits, petrochemicals in ground water supplies, industrial pollution in atmospheric air—is disease-causing and deadly. At the least **we see the causes** of sickness, systemic interference, organ malfunction and/or a series of periodic skin disorders, "ear infections," throat irritations, stomach upsets, headaches and a host of other, commonly known, 'drug store' and physician-dependent ailments.

But, none of these meet the strict definition of bodily "dis-ease" (or systemic disruptions which result from long-term accumulation of the interruption of normal bodily functions, especially metabolic elimination!).

As far as anyone can establish, *cancers*, perhaps the most feared of all "dis-ease symptoms (rivaled only by so-called "A.I.D.S."!) **have no single 'cause,' outside of the internal poisoning happening within the organism.** Surely, the general public is now convinced tobacco products ingested react with carcinogenic consequences on the body politic causing suffering, reduction in the quality of life, and premature death.

Alcohol claims more lives than do cigarettes; military and work place poisons claim their numbers as well. Polluted air and poisoned water, chemically altered and irradiated foods threaten the lives of more people than those replaced by the birth rate!

Thus, populations in 'developed' societies are diminishing while those in 'developing' societies are steadily increasing. This paradigm is what gives population issues their 'political dimension.' And, this demands we revisit the "AIDS pandemic!"

As a writer—and a lay 'social scientist' as well—viewing the larger picture differs, substantially, from that portrayed in the media, in schools, colleges and universities, and what is reflected in our culture, traditions and lifestyles in general. A cynic might conclude: **"There is a conspiracy to keep the people incapacitated and distracted by fostering confusion, misinformation and frustration!"**

I am persuaded by the science of Natural Hygiene, as researched and developed largely by Herbert M. Shelton, N.D. During more than a dozen years of studying and practicing a hygienic lifestyle, I have come to believe that **nutrition as we have been taught is a "false science" that is largely responsible for the range of so-called 'household' "diseases" already 'anticipated' by advanced preparations of over-the-counter-drugs, even before symptoms occur!** Of course, doctors and pharmacists 'know' these disease symptoms are forthcoming. It is clear to this writer that following the 'teachings and recommendations' of "nutrition" leads directly to the onset of disease symptoms. For example, children who never eat meat or drink milk just don't seem to ever suffer from "childhood diseases!"

Is Nutrition, as Taught, Incorrect?

If 'the idea of nutrition'—the notion that a 'certain balance' is most advisable for the 'proper growth and development' of the human species—is a noble concept, 'the science of nutrition' is, fundamentally, ignoble.

Therefore, an 'attack' on nutrition is like violating the innocence of a child, or defaming our national flag—like profaning the image of the Queen of England or bringing into ill repute the American notions of 'Motherhood and apple pie.' In respect of these delicacies, therefore, we will look, first, at what nutrition leaves out of its instruction—as to its 'errors and omissions.'

1. Is there anyone who is not unclear about the 'water issue?'
    a. How much water to drink each day?
    b. What kind of water (tap, distilled, spring, 'bottled,' filtered or 'gassed')?
    c. When should water be taken? Why?
2. Do you have unresolved questions about the 'protein issue?'
    a. Is it true, really, that humans 'need' animal protein to develop properly and to sustain ample 'building blocks' for those the body replaces?
    b. What, then of other protein sources: raw fruits, for example? Raw nuts and seeds? Grains and legumes? Green, leafy vegetables? Fresh fruits and berries?
    c. Is there really no 'cholesterol problem' Beyond Meat Eating? What of nuts?
3. Is there a difference between starches and carbohydrates? If so, what? If not, why not?
    a. Are there starches which our bodies more easily process and than others? Is starch made by man or by the Creator?
    b. If carbohydrates are natural, and fit for humans, are starches unnatural and, therefore, unfit?
    c. What of grains? Are they a recommended food for humans? Why? In what forms? Why or why not?
4. Are you clear about how much of any of the 'recommended nutrients' one should consume—and whether consumption should be daily as opposed to every third day, or even weekly?

a. How much is too much protein to consume? Is animal protein processed by the body differently from plant protein? Which, then, is better for humans?

b. Since animals do not drink milk after they are weaned, and so many of them are bigger, stronger and live long than humans, why are humans "encouraged" to drink unlimited quantities of milk all our lives?

c. How much food should one consume at a meal? In what order? How many different types of food should be in the stomach at the same time? And, what is the effect of heat and cooking on the presumed nutritional content of selected foods?

5. How many times should we chew each mouth (full) of food? Should "new" food be added to partially chewed food already in the mouth? Why does it matter how well food is chewed? Or, how long should food remain in the mouth before it is swallowed?

a. Is there any scientific relationship between a person's overweight and his or her chewing pattern? Do all fat people 'roll and swallow' their food? And, do they too quickly drink too much water or liquid, and too frequently?

b. Do cardiovascular patients show an alarming common trait of not chewing their foods, of eating in haste, and of consuming large amounts of animal products?

c. If "developed" nations **over** eat and underdeveloped nations **under eat**, which pattern is more disease causing? Is overeating "nutritious" foods more life threatening than just eating non-nutritious foods?

There are many additional questions that are not resolved for us by traditional "instruction in nutrition." Even Ph.D.'s in nutrition pass on incorrect advice and information, just as do their counterparts in medicine, who recommend drugs based on "lab reports" or "other considerations" from those who manufacture or market the drugs; or clerics who dare not depart from or "tolerate" questioning the standard dogma of their religious persuasions; of politicians who advocate, in all public appearances, "the party line."

Nor is it necessary, or practical, for every individual to know the same amount of correct information. While soldiers need not know much of what the generals know, many more soldier deaths result from "ill-advice" than from "sound advice." True, being sworn to follow orders is different from relying upon generally accepted instruction received at the university. The effect is the same, nonetheless. Specificity of input determines the course of human lives. Because of this single fact—as has been upheld in courts of law and of conscience, **an individual need never surrender his or her unalienable right to refuse to follow an unethical "order."** In military engagements, a soldier is never obligated to rape women, murder children or take pleasures on the corpses of the dead. In religion, one is taught and expected to co-exist with other beliefs, even if allowed to believe "there is only one true religion." In medicine, a doctor is not compelled to remove the wrong organ, or to prescribe untested, unproven and dubious drugs. Nutritionists, similarly, are not charged for not "warning" against the over consumption of protein foods, or for not pointing out the dangers inherent in under chewing, or of negative consequences of drinking fluids at the same time as having meals!

"Preacher" Reflects the "Teacher"

The science of sociology has long demonstrated a human model that is reliable. If a child is raised lovingly, a loving adult emerges; if a child is raised hating, an adult who hates emerges. If a child is abused, an abusing adult generally can be predicted. If being fat or "pleasingly plump" was the childhood norm, it is likely to be the adult norm as well. **Children eat what adults around them eat**; children learn to trust and believe what adults around them believe and trust. We all tend to teach others from the pool of instruction we have received. In this sense, the "preacher reflects the teacher."

Why the "Science of Nutrition" Is Incorrect

Having established some common ground, let us move now to consider why **nutrition**, as it has been and is being taught, is fundamentally incorrect. First of all, however, let us complete the critical implication of the previous discussion: If the classical lessons in nutrition are not correct, then it follows that those who teach, those who learn and those who practice nutritional "rules" must re-learn what is true and correct—into the next Millennium. That is the critical task for today, by ethnic groups (peoples with melanin) <u>killing themselves off more rapidly by their misinformed consumptive lifestyles.</u>

Four or Five "Basic Food Groups?"

The essential assumption or conclusion in the "science of nutrition" is that proper growth and development in humans (starting in infancy) relies upon "an adequate amount" (RDA, recommended daily allowance) of certain "elements" in foods, and that these "essential nutrients" are best derived from four or five groupings of food substances: 1-(animal) protein, 2-(manmade and natural) <u>starches-carbohydrates,</u> 3-<u>fruits and vegetables</u>, 4-<u>grains</u>, and 5-<u>sprouts</u> (considered by some). But, how were these four or five groups arrived at, you might ask?

Imagine you were in attendance at a very large convention, of thousands of growers, sheep herders, pig farmers, cattle ranchers, chicken farmers, crop growers, fishery growers, chemical manufactures, fertilizer producers, bottled drinks representatives, milk and cheese people, bakery goods representative, oil and butter producers, and advertisement executives—all with their lawyers and accountants. Can you think of anyone who would be left out of the "four basic food groups" formula?

That "nutritional science" is all-inclusive is not the critical issue, really. And, the important concern is one of relativity.

Reflecting upon that hypothetical convention you attended, now ask yourself: "Of all that I saw and heard—and was told to believe and trust—what, among it all, is absolutely the best for human growth and development?" Now comes our focus on the essential issue: reliable information.

"Nutrition" Is Not Reliable

Nutrition, as we have been and are being taught it, **is unreliable**. Animal protein, consumed by animals with very short and simple digestive tracts (intestine), is not a good food for humans (with our long—ten times body length—complex digestive tracts). Since humans, obviously, can live and seem to do quite well consuming animal fats and proteins, what seems to be the problem? **Excellent question!**

When animal protein must travel the length and complexity of the human digestive system, the journey will take days, not hours (as 'nutrition' allows us to assume). Slow-moving and putrefying (rotting) day by day, gases and toxic poisons are released into the human organism. So-called "bad breath" is just one symptom of the decaying process. Foul-smelling gas is another indication of internal decay going on. Over time, the build-up of these gas and chemical residues (at least their impact) and toxic waste matter, are debilitating, both to body functions and to body organs.

Ever wonder why the pharmacist or chemist can already know our "medical distress" and have the "prescribed" drugs and chemical formations ready and waiting for us when we arrive? Back to "the convention" for another reference: when the "delegates" left the convention, all left with smiles on their faces, because their interests had been served. **They had been assured a fair share of the consumer market or of what and how you and I would be taught to consume.**

And, as surely as healthy mother's milk protects and fortifies a healthy child with the stuff of good health, cow's milk assures the child a life of 'common childhood diseases' and "normal occurrences," such as the so-called "common cold," occasional high temperature (fever), ear-nose-throat infections, body rashes, and the rest.

What nutrition does not know—at least does not tell us—is that any disease is a direct effect (result) of previous and various "causes," our pattern of consuming food and drink being a major cause; our way of exercising, resting, and believing is another. More importantly, what we observe and react to—as with the "common cold"—**is** the evidence, for us to see, that an essential organ cleansing activity is required and is underway. This is true, as well, where there is pain or skin rashes. As most of the writers referenced in this volume attest, raising a child by the "principles of nutrition" practically **guarantees** the child will grow and develop through the series of sicknesses and diseases we refer to as "childhood diseases."

The fact is, however, disease conditions are not necessary to childhood, just as those we attribute to adults are not necessary to adulthood. "The proof is in the pudding." Evidence is abundant—though, understandably, not well publicized—that **children not raised on cows' milk, and who do not get "vaccinations" almost never come down with so-called "childhood diseases."** The record is not perfect, or absolute, because while parents may not allow the above, they might indulge the child with impure water, polluted air, drugs (medications), chemicals, or contaminated foods.

On the other hand, adults who follow a "wholistic" regime, and implement into their lives most of the 'Rules of Wellness' (Anderson, 1986) advocated by the **Organic Wellness Crusade Foundation** (P.O. Box 7219, Beverly Hills, California 90212-7219), this writer and others, seldom fall victim to such debilitations as heart disease, cancer, diabetes, stroke, asthma, hay fever, arthritis, organ failure, aneurysm, blood clot or other maladies. Of course, as with the consumptive patterns of children, other ill-advised consumables can bring about any other or the above disease conditions, as well.

For example, those vegetarian and wholistic practitioners in the Vietnam War who were exposed to "Agent Orange" (compounds of the nitrate chemical compound, "dioxin") were as seriously poisoned, but not more so than meat eating, nutrition-instructed individuals. Those from all participating countries who spent time on the front lines in the Gulf War have long since showed signs of "new and unknown" disease conditions (after ten years of 'denials' now referred to as "Gulf War Syndrome!"). However, those bodies which were plant fortified dealt better with the impact of the poisoning (whether from chemical weapons or from 'protective injections') than did the bodies that relied upon fortification from their animal-based diet. And while convincing statistically sound data to prove this conclusion were not available earlier on (because of so much denial, cover-up, misinformation and false mental constructs), it is reasonable to conclude that if the housekeeper arrives at your home directly from her own, she is better equipped or capable of cleaning your house than if she came from having already cleaned your neighbor's house that very same day! The point is that the "immune system" is weakened by the Standard American Diet (SAD). So, when crises come—whether stress or physical challenge—the plant-diet body is better able to cope than is the meat-diet body.

Summary Thoughts on 'Nutrition'

1. Sufficient "alternative" scientific evidence exists to question the reliability of the principles and precepts of nutritional science, as we were and are being taught. Therefore, colleges and universities must revise what they teach, or continue to be indicted by human experience, as the "foot soldiers" of those "generals" who derive their fortunes from what and how people consume.
2. The individual has the unalienable right to make choices that lead to healthful living—once he or she can access reliable information. And, while longevity cannot be guaranteed from recommended consumptive lifestyles alone, one can reasonably expect to escape falling victim to catastrophic disease conditions later in life, or to pain and

sickness in the earlier years. Thus, the payoff is much higher quality of life than is delivered by adherence to conventional nutrition.

The Standard American Diet (SAD)—acknowledged as being a departure from "the recommended daily allowances" as espoused by nutritional science, nonetheless, is recognized—even by the medical establishment—as a number one cause of ill health in Western society. In fact, "diet recommendations" by the physician are used, not to 'cure' the ailment, but rather to enhance the physician's 'status' as a concerned professional. **The simple truth is, concern about cholesterol is generally resolved by totally discontinuing the consumption of animal products!**

In short, this writer's pessimism—highly out of character, I might add!—stems from the realization that all these words describe but one simple truth: **how we eat, drink, exercise, rest, and think earlier in our lives, pretty much determine our quality of living later in our lives.**

According to Dr. Vetrano, "Young people who only care about the here and now and could care less about their bodies or health in the future should embrace this book, especially for admonitions on how we eat, drink and think. They are living for momentary thrills, completely blind or refusing to listen or even think that their lifestyles are guaranteeing them a future poor quality of life (the least of the results that are to come)!

This construct is so simple, yet so profound. The responsible choices given to us by Our Creator, through "free will," encourage either (a) being in charge of controllable factors or (b) declaring early on a disinterest in the later consequences in our lives. In short, to truly be responsible—emancipated from the manipulations of 'special interests'—one must (1) care enough about wellness principles to implement them into one's life, or one must (2) accept a come-what-may-attitude, and let society provide for a 'diseased older person' should you be so unlucky as to live to a ripe old age!

The rationalized 'compromise' to the above two options is what most people might be comfortable with*: the belief that "a cure will be found" and "my doctor knows best...!"*

Chapter One

Seminar with College Co-Ed's

(An informal 'seminar' of "wellness concerns that come to mind." Participants—all college co-ed's—are identified by age and sex only. In this manner, the reader is better able to relate to the unique contexts of the participants. The author believes this open-ended exchange maximizes honesty, and brings the reader passionately close to truth, 'hard truth' to end 1999 and to begin Millennium 2000!)

Summarizing the tenets of Natural Hygiene, isolating key perspectives from *The Nature and Purpose of Disease: Definitive Guide for Peoples with Melanin*, and invoking, 'the heart of T.C. Fry' and others, this writer laid himself out before a group of young people in Ikeja, Lagos, at the home of Nigerian publishers, Otunba (Dr.) and Chief (Mrs.) Victor O. Vanni. Participants were invited to ask any question on wellness 'that came to mind.' What follows is what occurred.

Male, age 26: Does Natural Hygiene believe in herbs?

Anderson: No, not really. Natural Hygiene holds that if one substantially meets the body's needs by eating foods of its biological adaptation, and indulges rest, sleep, sunshine, pure water, fresh air, exercise, warmth, tranquility and the 'fellowship of kindred spirits,' one will never be sick or diseased, and therefore would have no need for herbs or anything else.

Female, age 22: Why don't medical doctors live longer?

Anderson: I believe their use of their own 'medicines,' even to the level of addiction, is a contributing factor. As you know, doctors spend long hours, often without sleep or rest, sometimes for a few years or more on end. This is very taxing on the body;

it creates many hardships or crises for both organs and functions. A doctor told me he once worked 15 hours per day for seven straight years; and at age 49, he already could 'pass for' 69.

John H. Tilden, M.D., a physician for 67 years who followed more the ideals espoused by Natural Hygiene and discontinued "medicating his patients," described the "exhaustive expenditure of nerve energy" as ***enervation.*** When a body is 'enervated,' and remains so for too long, death is often a consequence. Some who intimately knew Dr. Herbert M. Shelton, "the father of Natural Hygiene," believe that he died from being too long enervated, at the time of his death being 'pushed' to complete yet another volume.

So, I would say the principal factor in the abbreviated life span of doctors is enervation.

Female, age 24: If cancer runs in a family, does that mean several of the women will get it, or several of the men, whichever?

Anderson: This is a good question and I know how important it is to many, many people. Let me approach my answer in this manner: The medical profession makes a big thing of "family history." The implication is always a negative one. If you have cancer in your family—or heart disease, or diabetes, whatever—you are more likely than others 'to be afflicted' by the same ailment yourself. If there is no cancer in your family history, no one ever says, "You are not likely to suffer from the disease of cancer because it does not run in your family!" Isn't that kind of curious?

Truth of the matter is that the only "family history" that impacts one's state of wellness, or his or her connection to disease, is "social history" or "social heredity." That is to say, mainly dietary shortcomings, combined with other violations of our natural requirements, conspire to cause and/or repeat the occurrences of similar diseases in people (family members) who engage the same bad habits. In short, people in the same family who 'come down with' the same diseases always "eat from the same table." The same bad habits beget the same bad consequences. This is borne out when we consider that the "black sheep of the family" almost never comes down with the "family diseases."

Do you see my point? Since drinking coffee (consuming caffeine) contributes to heart disease, a non-coffee (soda, tea, etc.) consumer will not have this 'negative' to deal with no matter how many others in her/his family did the opposite. John Harris, at Cottonwood Health Spa in Dothan, Alabama put it this way: "If you keep on doing what you've been doing, you are going to keep on getting what you've been getting." This applies to individuals, or to groups of individuals who engage the same punitive behaviors.

No, "family (medical) history" is never a factor in what disease/s any family member/s might experience. But, 'social history' is a critical factor. Unless the children change those negative behaviors of their parent/s, the children can look forward to suffering the same health conditions later in their own lives.

Male, age 25: Does the manner of cooking have anything to do with the quality of food?

Anderson: Yes, cooking (heating above 130F) kills the enzymes in food, produces chemical compounds, denatures the food and turns what might have been wonderful fruits, vegetables, nuts, seeds, grains and legumes into carcinogenic fare that is the foundation of cancer within the body politic. Boiling is better than roasting, baking better than frying, but 'slightly steaming' might be superior to any cooking method. What is eaten is, of course, a critical consideration.

Female, age 21: What about fish and meat?

Anderson: According to the research, empirical evidence and avocation of Natural Hygiene, the human organism is not anatomically designed to consume flesh foods. Humans are fundamentally 'vegetarians,' even fruitarians—physiologically structured to thrive on fruits, vegetables, nuts and seeds, organically grown and eaten uncooked primarily. Flesh foods remain too long within the human body, causing putrefaction and chemical reactions that poison the system (piecemeal) before the toxic stuff can be eliminated by body processes.

Meat eating animals have very short intestinal tracts for quick processing and elimination; or as in the case of certain serpents, provide for a long, slow digestion without causing internal harm. Not so with humans! The longer anything remains in the human organism the more deadly it becomes!

Flesh eating, in the West (and to a rapidly growing extend in Japan and other countries that adopt "the Western style of eating") is believed to be the leading cause of heart disease, the number one killer of adult Westerners!

In fact, most of the "feared and deadly diseases" like cancer, stroke, diabetes, arthritis, osteoporosis and even multiple sclerosis have their genesis in the consumption of flesh foods, cooked and containing 'animal fat' or "problem cholesterol."

I tell university students that drug stores exist, with their ready to use products, because eating the way we have been taught to eat (the "basic four food groups"), druggists can just sit and wait—just as can physicians—because "they just know that we are coming!"

Female, age 23: How long should a fast last?

Anderson: What I refer to as an 'organic, hygienic fast' (abstaining from all food, taking in only pure water) should last for three days, more or less, or until the body has resolved your issue; but, more importantly the fast should be ended on liquids (fruit/vegetable juices or broth/soup) one day for each three days of abstinence from "solid foods."

The ultimate length of time of a fast should relate to the purpose of the fast and disappearance of 'symptoms.' In other words, since fasting is a body-generated detoxification opportunity, which eliminates unwanted 'stuff' through the lungs, kidneys, skin and other organs, fasting should end when evidence of elimination ends, but well ahead of starvation.

Dr. Vetrano cautions, however, that "even though the symptoms disappear, if you do not go further, or as long as possible, the chronic disease resurfaces after the fast."

Female, age 21: When animals are sick, they stop eating; do you recommend people do the same?

Anderson: Fasting is the principal 'healing mechanism' ordained in Nature. When a 'dumb' animal, on the African savannas or in the bush, on a Georgia farm or in a California household, feels 'sick,' that animal will not eat food! Instead, it finds a quiet place to remain warm and rest until it feels better. When a deer breaks a leg, it finds a warm place to rest, abstains from food, and permits the bone to re-calcify, thus mending itself naturally. All other healing best takes place in the same manner, because <u>all healing is an innate body process!</u>

In other words, only the body can heal itself. The big task for humans is to not interfere! I cannot over-emphasize the role of fasting in the healing process; nor can I over emphasize the importance of "supervised fasts," in the care of wellness professionals trained in the art and science of fasting. Even a healthy body can be quickly poisoned to death. Fasting cannot prevent lethal injections, nor can it restore a spent organ. But it can help restore wellness to an enervated, toxic body.

Female, age 23: If there is nothing wrong with me, should I fast? And for how long?

Anderson: The first meal of the day gets its name, "break-fast" from our having fasted from sleep time to morning or awakening. Any period of time during which one or more meals are deliberately foregone, in the interest of body detoxification, shows appreciation for the body's natural needs.

Healthy people maintain their wellness through fasting to "prevent" toxic build-up. Twice a year, I will fast for not fewer than 7 to 9 days. My longest fast was 30 days, next longest 24 days, and none fewer than three days.

Female, age 21: If I go on a fast I can't do sports or anything else, can I?

Anderson: Perhaps you are not aware, prizefighters generally do not take any food on the day of their fights. Many cross-country runners do the same, and football players, and others. So, obviously, the answer is "Yes." You may still do sports while fasting.

Male, age 19: Does fasting mean you are starving yourself? And, why aren't starving people getting better?

Anderson: Excellent question! And, provocative! Fasting is not starving, even though in both cases the subject goes without food for long periods of time. The difference is during fasting the body draws on its 'reserves' or the nutrients stored as "fat."

When all these reserves are consumed, then—and only then—is the body undergoing starvation, for now it begins "to eat itself." The human body is largely protein and water. Breaking down self-protein is not poisonous to us. It is done on a daily basis even when we are not fasting. Animal protein is a deadly poison, because it putrefies before the body can dispose of it.

Male, age 23: When you have disease acting on the heart, kidney, etc. and you go to the hospital, they give you 'shots' or injections, medications and other treatments. Do you recommend taking what they offer?

Anderson: Try to avoid the hospital and call your Hygienic doctor first. But, when you are in such a poor stage as to be confined in a hospital, you might have little choice but to do as you are told! A wellness lifestyle may have prevented your having to go in the first place.

Female, age 21: Are you saying we all should become vegetarians?

Anderson: As I have said elsewhere, I believe human beings are vegetarians by anatomy and physiology, and in their pristine past ate only vegetables, fruits, nuts, berries and seeds.

Long human intestinal tracts, some ten times body lengths, all support the notion that vegetables do not generate the poisons that flesh generates when passing through the same systems. Vegetarians hold most of the Iron Man athletic records; vegetarians are less sick and experience radically fewer diseases than flesh eaters; and, vegetarian children seldom "come down with childhood diseases."

Female, age 23: I only have a bowel movement once every 4 or 5 days, and it has been this way since I was a child. Is that bad?

Anderson: Yes, it is bad; you're lucky you don't have asthma!

Male, age 24: She does have asthma!

Female, age 23: I do suffer from asthma.

Anderson: Well, I am not surprised. There is much evidence in hygienic literature that shows a direct correlation between asthma and infrequent bowel movements. In fact, there is strong evidence that cancer 'victims' also tend to experience less frequent intestinal elimination. And, this is consistent with what we have been saying*: the longer 'stuff' remains within the human organism, the more damage it causes* (from putrefaction or rotten protein).

But, your condition can be corrected by correcting your eating pattern. You need more fiber in your diet, less starch and less sugar; you need a diet of mostly raw fruits and vegetables, with some raw nuts and seeds of your liking. I think if you adopt the Natural Hygiene way of eating, and take care of the other body needs as well, you will find—perhaps in a shorter period than you ever dreamed—your stools will become more frequent and you will experience less and less discomfort from asthma. In fact, depending on how well you modify your consumptive behaviors, you can probably expect to be rid of the asthma altogether. Would that please you?

Female, age 23: I am going to do it! You will see: I am going to do it! Can I see you when you are back in the country?

Anderson: Yes, of course. I look forward to hearing your 'good news.'

Female, age 22: How can I gain weight?

Anderson: The recommended way, of course, is through exercise. 'Healthy weight gain' comes from increased muscle mass, as opposed to 'water weight' or stored 'body fat.'

Male, age 21: Is beer healthy?

Anderson: No, beer contains as much alcohol as does wine. When I travel in others countries, I can generally buy bottled water or pure watermelon juice, as is sold in Mexico. Carrot juice and the juices of many fruits, and vegetables are also available.

Male, age 22: Is palm wine good for you?

Anderson: Palm wine is perhaps on the order of vinegar, that is, it is partially fermented and as such provides welcomed atmosphere for the reproduction of certain bacteria. As a form of alcohol, it is no less detrimental once inside the organism. In short, palm wine is an alcoholic beverage, and all alcoholic beverages are compounds of sugar, resulting from fermentation, making them both 'addictive' and carcinogenic. In short, all forms of alcohol are poisons, and therefore are not recommended in a wellness program.

Female, age 21: I have read that "alcoholism" is a disease; is that correct?

Anderson: In a sense, but there is much more to it. In the first place, let me remind you that what we call "disease" is really dis-ease in the body; and dis-ease always results from some causative action or actions. In other words, as in the case of diabetes, consuming too much simple sugar (depleting the body's capacity to produce insulin) is NOT the ***cause,*** but one of the enervating factors. Toxemia is the cause; and diabetes mellitus is the result—the ***effect***, or what we call the disease.

I was brought up to believe—you no doubt as well!—that "a disease" was something you "caught." If you walked into a room where a number of people had common cold symptoms, you stood a pretty good chance of "coming down with a cold!" What we believed then—and most people still do! —is that we were 'exposed' to "other people's germs," and became sick (without 'cause'). That is how we were taught: that colds were one of the "contagious diseases" that periodically afflict "innocent" individuals.

The truth is, ***dis-ease*** is as "contagious" as is an accident (which **is always caused!**), whether intentionally or not! Once we come to grips with the Universal Law of "cause and effect," and apply its *rigid principle* to our everyday lives, we can no longer claim to be 'victims' of germs, "viruses," bacteria or any combination of "contagious substances." We come to understand that if the body is poisoned to the extent it cannot safely survive at that level of dis-ease, it will, of its own innate intelligence, implement processes (symptoms) to rid itself of the abundant toxicity. Usually, it will institute a fever, or boils, or skin rashes, mucus in the lungs, discharges, tumors and other strategies to isolate or capture, then discharge from itself the excessive poisonous material. This is how the "innate healing process" really works.

Female, age 24: Are you saying the alcoholic is responsible for his/her condition?

Anderson: Yes, definitely. But, the picture is larger still. The real "dis-ease" or cause is not alcoholism, in my judgment, but rather "addiction." Addiction is the consequence of consuming 'stuff,' which provides no nutrients or other useful ingredients for the body, but leech from the body its vital substances. Strange as it may seem when alcohol, drugs, caffeine, or even sugar is withdrawn from the body, this sets up a 'craving,' in some instances so great that "it takes control of mental and physical processes." This is why it is so easy to classify 'alcoholism' as "a disease condition." The bodily damage from wasting nerve energy processing "the stuff, and the enervation and nerve irritation cause the withdrawal symptoms," Dr. Vetrano reminds us.

The real dis-ease is **addiction**. In our society, children get started on the road to "addiction," which is really stimulation very early in life, usually with candy and ice cream—yes, and cake (especially 'birthday cake'). The 'addictive personality' is a misnomer; what we have in our society is a sugar-based lifestyle, which fosters 'addictions' of various kinds among all the people.

What we hear most about are the *relatively few* members of society who actually 'graduate' to addiction of more infamous substances, such as cocaine, heroin, sleeping pills, prescription drugs, so-called 'designer drugs,' herbs, vitamins, condiments, alcohol and all other forms of simple sugar (as in honey, bread, cakes, cookies, candies, flour, most cereals, beverages soft drinks and even filtered "fruit" juices).

Far more people lose their good health and their lives from sugar consumption than from cocaine consumption! The problem is, they do not know what is curtailing their well being and is causing their lowered quality of life, increased suffering and premature death! Just look, for example, at how much simple sugar is served as "refreshments" in churches and other community activities! Chocolates are deadly, but they are peoples' favorites, in many countries.

The fact that some people enjoy long lives, and many with relatively good quality, should not encourage 'rationalization' that sugar, or caffeine, or medications or drugs, or alcohol is any less deadly when consumed!

Alcoholism is one type of addiction; addiction is dis-ease in the body. Addiction results from counter productive actions by the individual, who is ultimately responsible for his or her "disease."

Female, age 24: I read your book (**Helping Hand: A Guide to Healthy Living, Beverly Publishers, Ikeja, Lagos, 1992**). I cannot eat what you recommend because we don't have those foods here (in Nigeria). So, what do you say to people in other cultures?

Anderson: First, I don't agree that you don't have foods to eat, which are recommended by Natural Hygiene. Every culture on the face of the earth has access to fruits, vegetables, nuts and seeds. Granted the diet of Eskimos is more animal protein than it is plant life; but Eskimos pay the price, too. They die relatively early, in their forties (apparently from the excessive protein, and the resulting taxation on the kidneys). But, in most populated areas of the world, it **is** possible to secure sufficient fruits, vegetables, nuts and seeds to maintain a 'vegetarian lifestyle,' and that's certainly true here in Nigeria!

Female, age 19: Do you recommend fasting for children?

Anderson: Actually, I don't have to recommend fasting for children. Children are still so close to their pristine beginnings, children will fast, automatically, when they are not feeling well! What happens is that parents tend to 'force' food onto children. If left alone children would fast a day or two, and recover quite rapidly from any temporary 'over-toxicity' and "be back to normal" in no time.

Male, age 26: The theory of fasting actually goes against all we were taught, doesn't it?

Anderson: Not totally. Some of us grew up in households that provided "chicken soup" when we children were ill. I remember my grandmother offering "a little broth" to one who was sick, and the admonition to "Stay in bed and rest yourself!" But, for the most part, you are correct: People who understood or believed in the principles of Natural Hygiene did not raise us. They did not know these principles, therefore they could not have taught them to us.

Now, the blessing is you and I can learn about these things and teach them to our children. In that way, the next generation will be better served.

Female, age 22: While away at school I became sick with typhoid, and I did not feel like eating. Health personnel told me I was weak because I needed to eat. Were they correct?

Anderson: Absolutely not! Your body told you it did not want any food; and that is what was correct. Not eating was far better for you than anything you might have eaten!

Male, age 20: You said malaria fever is the body attempting to heal itself; but doctors say malaria is caused by mosquito bites. With is correct?

Anderson: Malaria is the result of an increased number of parasites entering one's system; and the mosquito carries these. However, the accompanying fever is a body process, which is initiated to reduce the number of parasites, and restore the body to 'normality.' Generally, fasting and rest are adequate to deal with the average "bout of malaria." Your 'common malaria attacks' are about the equivalent of 'common cold attacks' in the

United States. Both can be 'treated' by abstinence from food and by resting.

Male, age 26: You talked about eating, but not much about other things like sleep. How much sleep is enough?

Anderson: "Eight hours" is the standard answer. The truth is, different people 'require' different amounts of sleep. One should sleep long enough to feel 'well rested' upon awakening. As I implied, for some people just four hours are what they need; others will require ten hours.

The wellness lifestyle advocated and promulgated by Natural Hygiene—and, therefore, by me—includes, consuming fruits, vegetables, nuts, and seeds, **uncooked** and **organically grown**; rest; sleep; exercise; sunshine; peace and quiet; warmth; friendly environment; pure water; clean air; positive thinking; laughter; the association of kindred spirits; and "not poisoning yourself," as in taking drugs or medications, consuming caffeine, sugar, alcohol, condiments and other poisonous substances.

Female, age 20: You've talked a lot about Natural Hygiene; how does one become a Natural Hygienist?

Anderson: One becomes a Natural Hygienist when one studies, learns and implements the principles of Natural Hygiene as the main features in one's lifestyle. Before an organizational "coup d'ete," one could join the American Natural Hygiene Society; but that option no longer exists. Even so, membership alone does not make one a Natural Hygienist. It's like people who join a Christian church, for example, and people who live a "Christian life." Which one is really the 'Christian?' I think you will agree it is the one who lives the life.

Male, age 18: Earlier, you spoke about fasting. If I don't eat, I feel hungry. How do I deal with 'feeling hungry?'

Anderson: What you 'feel' is not hunger, but "withdrawal pangs" associated with 'addictive' qualities in the regular food fare that you consume.

Male, age 18: I think I know—and I think everybody in this room knows—what hunger feels like. How can you say it's "addiction" withdrawal we feel?

Anderson: That is fair come back! Let me put it this way: A cleansed, detoxified, or hygienic body experiences a mild sensation of 'a need for food and/or drink.' There is no 'craving,' no desperation, and if elected, eating can be postponed without serious mental or physical disruption, and little or no consternation.

"The feeling of hunger," by contrast is a griping, sometimes painful, agonizing, and compelling sensation, which can drive some individuals to commit unspeakable acts! This is similar behavior to the 'withdrawal' experienced from nicotine, caffeine, alcohol, drugs, medications, sugar and many of the addictive substances we have spoken of during the evening.

Male, age 26: How can we as young adults design wellness lifestyles, when all we've been taught goes the other way?

Anderson: Well, once we have reliable information, 'designing' a wellness lifestyle is but a matter of choice and implementation. However, as is implied in your statement, how does one learn the difference between what leads to wellness and what leads to all the diseases in the book?

Obviously, at some point one must learn what is true—at least according to Natural Hygiene. And, there are others, not necessarily calling themselves Natural Hygienists, who advocate fundamental wellness principles that lead away from sickness and disease, drug free. Two such people are the late Dr. Alvenia M. Fulton formerly of Chicago, Illinois, and Dr. Bernard Jensen of Escondido, California. And, there are many others.

Female, age 24: Do you believe in a "conspiracy theory?"

Anderson: Yes, I do. Although I am not certain of your particular reference, I believe encouraging people to believe they "catch" somebody else's sickness is a conspiracy, to control and to manipulate. I believe what is taught in the university, as "the science of nutrition, namely the 'four basic food groups' is a conspiracy which guarantees future sickness, fosters the use of drugs and medications, and leads to the 'degenerative diseases' people experience later in life. I believe not telling people that "cancer" is the result of poisons stored, which mostly were consumed as foods and beverages, is a huge, profitable conspiracy! This ignorance keeps people dependent upon "medical therapies and scientific research" (at a cost of hundreds of billions of dollars worldwide!).

I believe telling school children—their teachers and their parents—to "Just say no to drugs" is a conspiracy to advertise drugs, drug usage and the availability of drugs, while giving the impression that the 'campaign' is some kind of "drug-use prevention" effort. Not so!

And, lastly, on this issue, I believe what might become the world's most profitable 'medical conspiracy' is what Dr. T.C. Fry refers to in ***The Great AIDS Hoax!*** Molecular biologist, Professor Peter Duesberg, at the University of California, Berkeley, California, has proven irrefutably, for example, that so-called *"HIV cannot cause AIDS because it is present in only half of the incidents of AIDS!"* Despite this scientific proof, speeches, publications and public discussions, those who control the media still have their high paid "news readers" telling the world everyday: "...HIV, the virus that causes AIDS!" That "big lie" is a big conspiracy! I also believe governments "conspire" to keep the truth from the people, in some cases, because the people do not want to know, and in other situations because people "cannot handle the truth!"

Female, age 22: Does fasting cause the stomach to go flat?

Anderson: Well, that could happen, depending upon the shape and size of the stomach to begin with and how long the fast lasts. The best way to flatten the stomach, though, is through vigorous, regular exercise and eating according to our biological adaptation.

The stomach is a pouch within the abdominal wall. During the abstinence from food, this pouch shrinks. What surrounds the stomach is abdominal fat. During a prolonged fast, the body consumes its stored fat. In many instances this means "a flatter stomach," from looking at a person's exterior.

Female, age 23: What can I do if I have asthma?

Anderson: Eliminating the intake of concentrated foods (like meat, fast foods, dairy products, soft drinks, and sweets) is a critical step. Eating lots of dietary fiber, as in raw fruits, vegetables, nuts and seeds, is another important step. Regular exercise will improve both digestion and elimination; and increased elimination is a critical factor in the life of an asthmatic. Rest and fasting should be done regularly, as well. ***First, though, I think one should arm oneself with lots of reliable information, as is found within the annals of Natural Hygiene,*** in books and papers written by individuals who daily maintain a lifestyle that is consistent with the principles of Natural Hygiene. Next, increase bowel movements—naturally—to at least twice each day.

Male, age 18: Is coconut a good dietary fiber?

Anderson: Coconut is readily available locally, I know; but it is not a highly recommended source of dietary fiber. Fresh vegetables, local fruits, raw nuts and raw seeds are the most highly recommended sources.

Female, age 21: What about garlic and onion?

Anderson: I have read that garlic, onion and lemon are three natural "antibiotics." As you know, Italians use a lot of garlic, and heart disease, among other things, is lower than in the West, but because of other healthful habits and not because of the garlic. Onion is often used in salads, and to a large extent to 'season' or influence the flavor of other foods. And, lemon has a variety of common uses, including use as a 'dressing' on raw vegetables and salads. However, both garlic and onions are to be avoided, as they are caustic and therefore negative dietary components. If you eat onions at all, use the sweet variety and not the "hot."

Female, age 23: Where can we (in Nigeria) find information about the principles of Natural Hygiene?

Anderson: Perhaps, the best source for reliable, hygienic information is any of a series of books authored by Dr. Herbert M. Shelton. Some university libraries might have one or more books by Dr. Herbert M. Shelton, Dr. Bernard Jensen, Harvey

Diamond, of course my own books, Michael Klapper, M.D., T.C. Fry, John H. Tilden, M.D., Dr. Hannah Allen, Dr. Alvenia M. Fulton, Dick Gregory, Adelle Davis and many others. Also, make use of the Bibliography in ***Helping Hand: A Guide to Healthy Living, and other volumes.***

I think that should be the last question. Thank you very much. I trust you have gotten as much from this sharing as I have. Good night.

Male, age 25: Professor, before we conclude, (one important question). Are you telling us that people—some of us know—who died of HIV or AIDS, did not have AIDS?

Anderson: Your question is very important, but not for the reasons you might think. A number of people have lost love ones; they've been told these loved ones died of "AIDS" (sometimes, because of family shame and embarrassment, its called "blood disease, pneumonia, kaposi sarcoma, or just plain, 'It!'"). The truth is many 'old diseases' have been lumped together and are called "AIDS." The point is all these 'causes of death' are drug related. No one ever died of "HIV or from any 'virus' of any kind!" But, what people believe is their only 'reality.' ***Until people face the truth that consumption of drugs and medications is killing their loved ones, they will continue to 'believe' such deaths are occasioned by "HIV, the virus that causes AIDS."*** That belief is simply not true! But, you should expect "the other guys" to persist in finding ways to keep you convinced that you are more 'at risk' from some mythical "virus" than you are from your involvement with drugs and chemicals. So long as people believe that lie, they will not and cannot wage a successful defense to protect themselves from the real culprits. What else can I say, but good night and thank you very much?

Chapter Two

The Words of T. C. Fry

The well-established and incontrovertible fact that humans are biological fruit-eaters arouses vehement objections from almost every dietary faction in America and the world including, of them all, those who will readily admit that we are fruitarians!

I have been a fruitarian (a predominantly eater of fruits) for the past 25 years. Even as a boy, in retrospect, for the first 16 years of life, I was a heavy eater of fruits.

In looking back, I now know that much of my "superiority" over students in my school and my ribbons won at curricular track meets were due to my heavy fruit-eating, my propensity for listening to classical music at every opportunity, being a "bookworm" devoted to mostly nonfiction books and excelling at games like checkers and dominoes.

My late love affair with fruits began in 1970 when I became a Hygienist. My innate fruitarianism reemerged and I've been a fruitarian ever since with my fruit intake being from 85% to, at times, 100% of my intake.

Here are a wealth of headlines which embody a cornucopia of revelations: "FRUIT-EATERS, BIG BRAINS! VEGETATION-EATERS, SMALL BRAINS! FRUIT-EATERS HIGH-ENERGY CREATURES! VEGETATION-EATERS LOW-ENERGY CREATURES! COWS' MILK A FAST-GROWTH, LOW-ENERGY AND SMALL BRAIN FOOD! HUMAN MILK A SLOW-GROWTH, HIGH-ENERGY AND BIG BRAIN FOOD! SMALL-BRAINED CREATURES NURSE FOR SHORT TIME IN NATURE! LARGE-BRAINED CREATURES NURSE FOR A GREAT TIME IN

NATURE! BIG-BRAINED CREATURES SLOW TO MATURE! SMALL-BRAINED CREATURES FAST TO MATURE! BIG-BRAINED CREATURES FAST-WITTED AND SMART! SMALL-BRAINED CREATURES SLOW-WITTED AND DULL!"

All this is derived from an article on the subject of vegetation-eating monkeys and apes compared with fruit-eating monkeys, chimps and humans.

In ***Discover Magazine*** for May 1995, there appears an article entitled "Gut Thinking," wherein its author, Peter Radetsky, presents the results of 20 years of study of primates (monkeys, chimps, apes and humans) by anthropologist Katherine Milton of the University of California, Berkeley.

The subheading is: "What makes fruit-eating spider monkeys so much smarter than leaf-eating howlers?" The article reflects that the fruit-eating spider monkeys had 107 grams of brain matter while the same sized monkeys, the leaf-eating howlers, had only 50.4 grams.

Moreover, the spider monkeys were highly energetic and moved a lot because fruits are fast-energy foods whereas the howlers were languid and slow because vegetation translates into very poor energy-yielding food.

Katherine Milton's closing observation is worthy of note: "<u>Everything comes back to diet</u>." It is the pivotal feature, the kickoff. When you get right down to it, the way we behave had better translate ultimately into groceries - - or we're not going to be around to behave that way much longer.

Dare I translate the obvious import of Dr. Milton's statement? She is saying that, "If you don't use it, you lose it!" If you do not exercise your disposition as a fruit-eater at the grocery counter, you become a dull-witted person! Eating a primarily fruit diet is the key to human intelligence, energy and virtues. We are the product of fruit-eating forebears. We should continue the tradition or sink into mediocrity.

Relationship between Diet and Disease

Most of today's foods cause sickness, diseases and cancer! Certain foods and their nutrients deliver resolute well being. For example, the "sickling" of red blood cells (where in the roundness is lost and a crescent shape results), makes it impossible for these oxygen-carrying cells to fold and enter into the gossamer thin capillaries, about 60,000 miles of which are in the average human body and causes severe pains at points where un-transported sickle cells accumulate.

A West African scientist, Dr. Oji Agbai, did extensive research on sickle cell anemia in the University of Arkansas Department of Pathology, Clinical Laboratory for Medical Sciences in Little Rock. He completed Ph. D. studies at City University Los Angeles, and in 1986 his findings were published in the Journal of the National Medical Association, Vol. 78, No 11.

He discovered that the sickle cell trait, an inherited defensive mechanism against malaria that was perfectly harmless, was on this order:

In many peoples of the world, not just Africans, the sickle cell trait exists in up to 50% of the population. In African Americans, 8% have this inherited trait. In Africa, 24% of the population has the same trait. [In Greece – 49% and in India – 32%]. In America, sickle cell anemia is suffered 20 times as frequently by those with the trait as in Africa!

Dr. Agbai learned that the incidence differential between Black Americans and Black Africans was attributed to environmental factors unknown and not understood. In researching these "environmental factors," Dr. Agbai came up with the answers.

He found that, just as anemia (meaning without blood) was generally caused by a deficiency in usable iron and vitamin B-12, so, too, sickle cell anemia was caused by yet another deficiency: thiocyanate. This compound is essential to healthy blood as cyanocobalamin is to the formation of vitamin B-12 that is also essential to healthy blood.

Dr. Agbai found that the Black African diet was heavy in thiocyanate-containing foods whereas their Black American counterparts ate precious little foods with this nutrient.

Dr. Agbai's solution to the problem was to feed Black American sufferers a diet rich in thiocyanate. Recovery was not relatively rapid, but as long as the diet was observed, permanent.

Foods known to have significant amounts of thiocyanate are lima beans, yams, cassava, cabbage, carrots, apricots, flaxseeds, broccoli, cauliflower, and peaches. Does that account for the fondness of most Black Americans for the most nutrient-dense food in the country, collard greens, a cabbage family member? Collard greens are rich in this and all nutrients except carbohydrates.

In my concluding comments, let me say: (1) the terrible statistics about diseases in America are caused in large part by the SAD [Standard American Diet] and pathogenic ways of life in America! (2) Neither the cells nor the body can be made "immune" to causative forces. The law of cause and effect can neither be suspended nor nullified! (3) Diseases cannot be prevented while their causes are in force. Diseases do not have to be prevented inasmuch as they will not happen unless caused!

Perhaps as important an illustration to the wisdom of Dr. Anderson's book lies in its implied refutation of the 'contagion theory.' "Viral attack" is a concocted myth. First, virii are dead and therefore inert. These genomic materials are derived from mitochondria that expired with the death of the cell of which they were a part. Genomes called virii (viruses) are the remains of the onslaught of the cell's disintegrative lysosomes released simultaneous to cellular death. Dead materials attack nothing! In the case of so-called cytomegalovirus, everything is the same except that the origin of a giant genome was the cell nucleus itself.

Finally, the 'secrets' which promise you need "never be sick again!" are buried between the pages of this volume. Your commitment to implementing living practices and purpose into your lifestyle only can be enhanced by ***The Nature and Purpose of Disease....***

—T.C. Fry,

THE WELLNESS NETWORK
Wellsboro, PA 16901
May, 1995

Author's Note:

Dr. T.C. Fry died September 6, 1996, as a result of unclear causes, shortly after a visit to an "ozone treatment facility" in the Dominican Republic. This volume is re-dedicated to his memory and legacy. For the essence of the man, see "Interview with T. C. Fry" (in this volume and at http://www.organicwellness.com)

Chapter Three

'Causing' Sickness and Disease

The nature and purpose of disease has confounded researchers and medical thinkers since the time of Imhotep, in Ancient Africa down through the Greek priest, Hippocrates, erroneously credited with being 'the father of modern medicine', and author of the Hippocratic Oath, even to the present generation.

The fundamental error is a historic one, an error of attrition. It is 'scientific' in that "science" is what prevails in its name. It is structured and systemic, between *then* and *now*, and hence to *the End.* The problem is: man has no capacity to know either the Alpha or the Omega, the Beginning or the End; man is a vain and arrogant creature who admits of no fallacies.

Through the ages, there have been periodic glimpses by a few. St. Thomas Aquinas acknowledged God, for example, to be "The Absolute…the First Cause," putting quite some distance or time between that absolute happening and any subsequent awareness known as the human time line. The Apostle Paul concurred when he taught, "We but see through a glass darkly…we know in part but when that which is whole is come…" Albert Einstein expressed the reality through physics and mathematics; establishing once and for all the relevant "sixth dimension" of human existence: *time*. But, even Einstein did not bother to argue the point of eternal or absolute time. Nor did he elaborate on the most essential dimension, consciousness.

Without consciousness, reality reverts to abstract existence or mere creation. Einstein was content with relative time as it reasonably could be calculated in relation to the speed of light. At best, he took human 'awareness' for granted.

The 'Age' of Disease

Disease is concomitant with the human species in its violations of the laws and principles that govern human existence. Despite human monopoly, disease is becoming characteristic of the universe itself. In other words, like other things "disease" in the consciousness of humans is also found in nature, affecting all existence. (1) This is because consciousness is energy, inclusive to the cellular level. (2) Constructive energy is (balanced), destructive energy has become 'unbalanced'. (3) Dis-ease is accumulated imbalance—an electrical dynamic. (4) All forms of manifest energy that predate the human species was then, is now and ever shall be subject to disruption of dis-ease, or to the random, predictable and unpredictable effects of the ever-continuing First Cause, paraphrased in the scientific community as the "Law of Cause and Effect."

But, how quickly the human species has forgotten the implications of St. Thomas Aquinas's admonition: <u>the First Cause is Absolute</u>. And, since the human race was not around at the very Beginning, there can be no human connection to that causal event. How this plays out for finite humans is as St. Paul said it: "We but see through the glass darkly; we know in part...."

Another look at the Law of Cause and Effect and we now can see absolutely nothing: for the assumed Beginning was beyond our consciousness and capacity to perceive, and the non-ending End postdates our consciousness. We have no ability to perceive that eventuality, either. What, then is the Universal Principle that governs human life and existence? And, does this principle also govern *the nature and purpose of disease*? Consciousness or Energy has its own properties, built-in principles—some known, most still unknown, and many that might never be known. There is, however, one probable 'universal principle,' extending even to other galaxies.

The Universal 'Law of Effects of "Cause"'

Within the limited scope of human capacity, there is "the need to know." It, however, is but a fantasy, a flirtation. It, like religion and drugs and sex and overeating, is a possessive delusion, an opiate. Perhaps, this is why so-called modern man moves human existence steadily towards extinction, while our ancient forefathers and foremothers, fore-cousins, especially those given to piety and meditation, were so attuned to the Universal Principle, even without being able to know its certainty.

The place of humans in the specter of existence is somewhere between the Beginning and the End if, indeed, there is a Beginning and an End. Yet, the Law of Cause and Effect implies only the Alpha and the Omega. Neither of these defines nor characterizes human consciousness. Therefore, our being is a finite existence, limited by time and capacity. So, it is delusion to think humanity can know that which is unknowable, whether at the Beginning or at the End.

'Perpetual Motion' Consequences

Therefore, what governs human existence might be called **"the Law of Effects of Cause."** Again, employing Einstein's demonstration of time, as a dimension of existence, one can reasonably say that eventualities after the Beginning are all Effects of Absolute First Cause. And having said that, we proceed immediately, to the conclusion that all human events are effects of Cause. This notion might be extremely upsetting to traditional intellectuals. It appears to incapacitate us.

Yet, there is consolation: all effects become 'causes' that lead to subsequent effects. Those effects which precede a particular eventuality may be—and often are—called "causes." Those which postdate the event are referred to as "effects." Thus, we get the non-scientific principle referred to as the "universal law of cause and effect." The law known as "the universal law of cause and effect" is a misnomer and is nonscientific because it is finite. The universal law of "effects of cause" is absolute; and, as we have already pointed out, human consciousness cannot perceive that which is Absolute. Consciousness, as energy, at the cellular level, is part of the universal 'absolute,' as we will see more clearly later.

Yet, if you have followed this line of presentation closely, it might by now be clear that our principle is, really, very simple: the existence of an Absolute Principle—call it God or Creation or First Cause or Allah or Unmoved Mover or Alpha or Absolute Spirit or The Creator or by any other designation—sets in perpetual motion subsequent eventualities.

Applying 'the Test of Common Sense'

These 'effects' can be observed, to a limited extent, by moving "backward" into an event: the birth of a child; the death of a pet; the crashing of an airplane; the murder of a person; the carnage of war; even the 'rage' of a tornado. With each of these eventualities, it is possible to "walk back into time," so to speak, a reasonable distance and observe some of the "causes" (pre-effects) of the particular eventuality (specific consequence or effect). A child is born because a woman has the biological capacity to nurture the fertilized egg. The egg is fertilized because, more than likely, a single male sperm was successful in penetrating the ovum. We have not yet looked at social aspects; nor at the conception of the male and female involved in this particular birth of this particular adult child!

A pet dies from 'cause.' But, the very 'cause' itself is the result (effect) of old age, trauma, or 'accident' and any of these are, surely, but effects of antecedent effects (causes). Likewise when a plane crashes. It is a resounding effect, stemming from all contributing effects, a limited number of which is uncovered through investigation. This backtracking goes only so far, however.

In a murder, as we are very aware, police look for "clues" to the murder. They look for method, means, opportunity and motive. They attempt to reconstruct "the events leading to the death of the victim." They gather 'evidence' to establish such things as time of death, type of weapon used, and the probable number of persons who might have committed the murder. Perhaps, this helps to explain why 'murder' is the most popular element in American drama!

Earthquakes occur—and sometimes produce tidal waves—depending on their location and force. Their seismic power comes from 'the build-up of pressures,' movement of earth formations, physiological and chemical activities, and a combination of factors. Efforts are made, after the fact, to ascertain the relative cause or causes of the earthquake, any tidal wave and/or the resultant damages.

There are no winners in war; yet, our selected memories do not permit us to 'remember' that old people and young children were killed during wars; that pregnant women and handicapped seniors were blown apart; that many people 'on both sides' died of shear fear and utter terror—of deathly fright! Yet, when the carnage is over both sides and all participants applaud their "heroes" and "heroines."

A tornado comes because the conditions were 'right' for it to come; and it moves in its own direction and with the destructiveness matching the contributory causes. It has no concern for humans or animals or property; and it gives no consideration to time of day or night, day of the week, month of the year or, for that matter, state or country, except as its own "causes" dictate. It is a thing that happens, the effects of prior "causes." Only so much can become known about these prior effects. Yet, when sufficiently studied, patterns emerge.

Not only is there limited capacity to continue to walk back toward First Cause, there is an unwillingness of humans to reach beyond their comfort zone—what we referred to earlier as the need to be deluded or "the need to know."

Believing What Is Not True

The tendency toward intoxication—whether strong drink or strong belief—is the human 'cover' for the wholesale inability to perceive the neutrality of eventualities. Unable to penetrate the Beginning or the End, humankind plays a game of "Let's pretend." So, we pretend plane crashes are "tragic," but war murders are "heroic." That the abortion of an unborn child is "sinful and cruel," while the starvation of a third of the world's population is "unfortunate, but political." Events are neither "good" nor "bad," whether "caused" by human greed—as we perceive it—or by "natural disaster." All events are effects of earlier causes, themselves the effects of the First Cause.

If a perfect state of health or wellness is the First Cause, then dis-ease, the less-than-perfect eventuality of human behaviors (pre-effects of 'cause') of a later condition or eventuality (effect), is preordained and is, therefore, incontrovertible. This is so not because of any preexistence of so-called virii but because <u>human consumptive afflictions and behavioral habits, patterns and actions beget "dis-ease conditions</u>."

This would make medical science at least partially, institutionalized fraud. And, all claims of "funding for research," or of "finding a cure" are but delusions, designed to appease a population which worships its own "need to be told something" (whether, in fact, what they are told is 'true' or 'false').

Many writers and researchers—truth seekers who stumbled upon fundamental and reliable 'truths' about the human condition, or who caught a glimpse of 'wisdom' in the exhortations or the lifestyles of zealots—have been, through the years, tormented that so close they seemed to have come to solving the human puzzle, only to be confounded later by their limited capacity to approach either the Alpha or the Omega of human consciousness. Rather than emancipate the people with truth, media campaigns ensnare citizens in lies shielded by created "institutions."

This dilemma is forever troubling. As we shall see as we go along in this writing, humans have a limited but sufficient capacity to perceive what is necessary to prevent disease in our lives; and, lack of perception in this sense, is not really the reason people experience disease. *The primary reason is that humans are encouraged to find more solace in believing what is not truth than in knowing what is true.* How many people will admit that "chocolate is not good for me," yet eat it anyway? How many know that smoking reduces the length and quality of life? Would you believe that drugs—medical, recreational and over-the-counter—are life threatening, debilitating and detrimental to health, wellness, longevity, happiness and quality of life?

Haven't you read 'research' that says margarine is 'not good' to consume, implying that butter is better? What of the coffee research, on the one hand castigating caffeine and on the other hand, pointing out the evils of decaffeinated coffee? And, who has not been confused by whether it is "all right" to eat eggs "four days a week" or "four eggs a week?" Who will dare question the constant promulgation that "milk makes a body strong?" What difference do you think it would make in the behavior of most people if they knew for certain, *none of the above is in the best interests of human well being?*

Perhaps the most serious threat to America's survival is a combination of the power exerted upon the people by the American Medical Association and the people's gullibility, particularly as related to *contagion* in general and the AIDS phenomenon in particular. The net result is that Western populations are 'conditioned' to such an extent, millions in Africa and Asia can be methodologically 'killed off' while we in the West attribute those deaths to "a deadly virus." To paraphrase William Shakespeare, this invention will live to plague its inventors.

Behaviors Beget Disease Conditions or Wellness

What we call disease is not a 'punishment' in a moralistic sense; it is, instead, a natural effect of 'causal behaviors' (our own and those of others!) It is a 'statement,' really, a statement that debilitating life-consuming practices have taken place. But, we already know the eschatological reason for what is referred to as the "onset of disease." What we now want to explore are more practical perceptions of *the nature and purpose of disease.*

According to Herbert M. Shelton, ND, disease is the result of bad intake behaviors, which are inconsistent with human physiology. Dr. Shelton points toward 'retained toxicity,' a phrase this writer finds useful. John Tilden, MD, practiced conventional medicine for many years, experimenting for a large part of some 67 years by administering to his patients a placebo, a purified water solution instead of expected medications. His patients experienced such an increase in healing, from all sorts and descriptions of disease conditions, Dr. Tilden permanently resigned from the practice of conventional medicine, spending the greater part of his professional years advising those who would listen concerning the real character of disease. He referred to disease as "a crisis of toxemia."

Perhaps one of the most learned researchers of modern times was my mentor, the late T. C. Fry, D.Sc. Not formerly "mis-educated" as Dr. Fry put it, "by conventional mis-education" but being self-taught, "T. C."—as he was affectionately called—referred to himself as "Mr. Fry," despite his honorary doctor of science degree from City University Los Angeles, and many other awards because he said, "I have developed a disdain for the term 'doctor,' as it is associated with those who misrepresent sickness and disease, both of which are preventable." Disease-free wellness, according to Dr. Fry, is accomplished by "an incredible diet...super delicious and super nutritious, yet is inexpensively available in your local super market the year around."

The physics or electrical aspects of organic fruits and vegetables, raw or at least not over- cooked, is the electrical charge of the foods and the resulting cellular balance created when such foods are consumed. When such foods are not the dominant diet, dis-ease at the cellular level results, giving rise to the many 'disease symptoms' known to us all.

Disease as a 'Thing' You "Catch"

Very often spoken of and written about as if an entity, or as a group of entities, disease and diseases are indelibly stamped in the human mind as "something you catch." Advocates of this notion rest heavily with both the medical community, who make their living from public responses to the notion, and the religious community, whose own financial well being is inextricably tied to the sense of "sin" or punishment for "wrong behavior." What tends to lull the public is that the notion is often reinforced, mixed with little truth and with much fiction, especially when advocated by 'celebrity' endorsers; who run, walk and even take off their clothes for certain "charitable causes."

The "truth," as has been often pointed out, reflects what all of us know: "The Absolute Law of Effects of Cause." Since the Absolute Rule has been established, concerning living life sickness and disease free, violations of The Rule result in sickness, disease, unnecessary and long term suffering, and premature death. But, this truth is too simplistic. It is aggravating, too, because it says, simply, "Drug use (recreational and prescription) results in A.I.D.S." But, I ask what need did Mother God, the First Cause, the Absolute One, Allah have to "impress" finite humans who would not even appear on the time line of existence until millions of years after the Absolute Rule was established?

'Role-Over' Effects

This is precisely why this writer submits that what best describes the human experience is "roll over effects." That is to say, every eventuality in human existence, whether 'experienced' or not, is [simply] another [inevitable] effect (of an earlier "effect"), which for human, finite purposes is called a "cause." In summary, "right eating, drinking, exercising, believing, and resting behaviors do not produce sickness and disease," but instead healthy, productive and happy lives.

From the perspective of Natural Hygiene, disease is often characterized as "not a thing, but a body process." This reference is not contrary to what has been offered above, but does expand our understanding. In this school of thought, which Dr. Tilden embraced, what is perceived as "disease" is but the dynamic and vital action of the organism to rid itself of the toxemia Dr. Tilden, Dr. Shelton and many others refer to as the "toxic condition" and what some lay people call a "caught ailment." Now, however, we are beginning to comprehend ***the nature and purpose of disease.***

Mothers with children are the most perplexed, and the most vulnerable because for them their ignorance could result in the untimely death of a child; and the public would be outraged! What panics them is the possible "effect" of death: They are not always aware of the misguided information and courses of action which, more often than not bring on the feared outcome. In other words, parents who teach meat-eating to their children, and who feed their children animal products including cow's milk, and who indulge inoculations and medications and "baby foods" in the lives of their children will experience so-called "childhood diseases," periodic sickness and occasionally the unfortunate death of an infant. Nor is it easy for parents. In some states still, parents who do not haul their infants in for poisonous injections are severely punished. Their children are often not allowed to attend public schools, for example, and worse this parent or these parents are blamed for "the spread of 'contagious diseases' among children."

People who consume so-called "ethnic-foods" are, very often the next most controlled group and, therefore, contribute most to their own demise. We understand the nutritional contents of ethnic foods tend to differ within and without regions and countries. Nevertheless, the fundamental sickness and disease-generating characteristics tend to be constant: high seasoning, animal products, over consumption, and little regard for the body's digestive, assimilative and eliminative needs. And, too often no concept of essential nutrients exists, nor of the ratio of one nutrient to another, in the overall scheme of human physiology. It is, in words T. C. Fry might use, "a travesty of mis-education."

By far the largest group of individuals who "consume themselves into disease conditions, unnecessary suffering and premature death" are those who consume the S.A.D. (Standard American Diet). The next largest group has a reasonable option, and those who—given the availability of reliable information—just don't seem to care about preserving well being, particularly when life is yet very vigorous! This latter group is committed to "preferred lifestyles." This is a fundamental decision. And, everyone has the God-given right to choose behaviors that lead to sickness and bring about the disease process. This is a most unacknowledged human right!

When confronted, however, with having "chosen" the "effect" which shall be theirs, people are quick to believe their past behaviors are unrelated to their disease conditions; that what really happened is they "caught somebody else's disease," and are themselves, "innocent" of any earlier "causes." Such people are quick to explain that "this or that disease is going around!" or "Brett has HIV, but don't know how he got it!"

Tell people, "You did not catch a cold, or the flu, or so-called 'HIV;' you brought it upon yourself, or someone brought the poisoning upon you. Your body is just telling you it is over toxic and needs to clean house," and they react as if you just insulted them. Of course, there are exceptions; and, the group which is most likely to make the exception is the final category of individuals for purposes of these illustrations.

People Who Care About Wellness

'People who care about wellness' (Anderson, 1986) make up only ten to fifteen percent of the overall population, according to Dr. T.C. Fry. Others are as indicated above: those who have 'other reasons' for not engaging behaviors that produce health as opposed to sickness and disease. Yet, it is to these relatively few that the science of Natural Hygiene must speak. It is for this group—even as it increases in size—that simple truths must be explained and examined, over and over again. **Proper behaviors must be articulated, so that the right behavior is not done in the wrong context, thus turning a positive into a negative.** The 'common sense test' must be constantly demonstrated, such that there is always a 'yard stick' by which to measure recommended consumptive behaviors. In the words of movie producer, Spike Lee, it is critical in wellness, too, to "do the right thing!"

All 'Diseases' Are the Same 'Disease'

What might strike some as 'shocking' is the contention that "all diseases are the same disease." In other words, all disease conditions are a single message: <u>toxic overload.</u> Therefore, that which resolves one disease condition will resolve all other disease conditions, even so-called "incurable diseases."

Why is this so, you ask? It is so because 'common sense' confirms it: behaviors—not compounds—that assist the body in cleansing any of its parts will cleanse all of its parts. So, a physiological rest, for example, will not only 'conquer' the flu in a person, but it will also 'consume' a tumor. A headache is eased by the same abstinence or fasting activity that enables the body to heal an ulcer. A detailed discussion of fasting comes much later in this volume. A change in wellness habits and behaviors improves one's vision. It also improves one's performance activities in other areas, including sexual fulfillment.

To the majority of medical practitioners, the above paradigms are "heresy!" Yet, these very physicians are known to quip, "Take two aspirins and call me tomorrow." In Natural Hygiene, we would say: "Take no food; go to bed and rest; and in one-to-three days you should be back to 'normal.'" And, it is fair to say that *an increasing number of conventional medical practitioners are backing off prescribing drugs for their patients'* every complaint. This is a positive trend with those calling themselves 'holistic' practitioners taking the lead.

Hygienic advice is, I believe, infinitely wiser and healthier than routine "medical advice." Hygienic counsel is so simple and inexpensive, most people do not give it the credence it deserves. It seems they would rather incur "costs" by having physicians tell them what is not true, what is less helpful, and what is infinitely more deceptive and dangerous in the long run. People not only pay hundreds of billions of dollars to physicians each year to hear, "You will live," but they as often pay hard earned money out and also submit to dubious procedures, just because "My doctor said so."

The 'Science of Nutrition' Has Been Debunked

College educated people are really the most "mis-educated about health." This is so because they learned to believe that which continues to fail 'the common sense test.' The stork never did, and never will deliver a baby; no tooth fairy ever exchanged a tooth under the bed pillow for a twenty-five cents piece. Saint Nicholas or Santa Clause never came down the chimney himself, let alone bringing the bicycle with him! If "Christ died for our sins," why isn't human experience now 'sin free?' Can you put your hand in fire, and have it burn your neighbor's hand? Can you "catch" a broken leg? Does the 'common cold' result from toxic overload and enervation, or from "a bug going around?"

Before we were taught 'the science of nutrition' in elementary, secondary and post secondary schools, we were fed according to our mothers' orientation. We were fed meat very early, as part of our 'baby foods' and in conjunction with 'childhood medications.' All this was done to us in the name of "health."

'Maturing adults' are a marketing threshold; the words mean consumers, sources of revenue and objects of the 'genius of Wall Street.' To understand the implications of what it is we are suggesting, you must remember the imaginary convention where everyone was invited, except you and me, the consumers. This convention took place sometime in the past. Imagine....

Dairy industry people came; meat, fish, poultry and egg people were there. Weight loss people sent their best brains, and so did the exercise equipment people. Fertilizer, insecticide, pesticide and chemical people were represented. Packing people, and advertising executives came. Beverage people—carbonated sodas, wine, beer, alcohol, coffee, tea, and even water bottling people were present. Sugar, sweeteners, food coloring, food preservatives and freezer makers came also. Wheat and bread people attended; hematologists and elixir mixers showed up; butter and cooking oil people were there; spice manufacturers and salad dressing makers came, too. Those who make cans, and those who make plastics were there. Of course, vitamin supplements people were represented. Vegetable and fruit growers also came. And nuts and seeds people. Dietitians and nutritionists were everywhere; so were gourmet chefs and ordinary cooks. Exotic food marketers were there as well. School superintendents and food dispenser people were there. Drug and pharmaceutical houses were there, and many from the medical profession. Religious people and psychics came early. In short, everyone you can imagine came to the "convention" and, everyone left out of the big hall with smiles on their faces. All the attendees got something conceded in their favor.

You and I did not attend the convention; we did not go because we were not invited. Yet, we were the subjects of all that took place. Attendees agreed among themselves: "You don't tell them what to eat; and we won't tell them what to drink!" Since then, in every restaurant and on every airplane, you and I might be asked, "What will you have to drink?" And the question is asked just as we are about to eat, the very time no drinking should take place! A deal was struck. You and I were sold out!

What emerged from that convention are the bases for most disease conditions, sicknesses and disabilities humans can be expected to experience in the course of their dubious lives.

The "four basic food groups" were established by those who attended the convention; and, our adherence to the 'dictates of nutrition' as it has been taught to us guarantees a life of sickness and disease. Some of the evidence of this simple truth can be observed at our local pharmacy, with already prepared drugs waiting for us to come and get them. And an army of "medical people" is fielding our visits and phone calls. Somehow, they seem to know we are coming! A word to the wise is therefore, appropriate: If you can read the "nutritional contents' of a food, avoid it! For, natural foods have no 'contents' labels.

What Other Choices Have We?

Realistically, before any of us have real choices, we must have reliable information (Anderson, 1986). This is what is missing from most television, print media, radio, interview and talk shows. What the public gets is the mass dissemination and reiteration of misinformation! How serious is it? Not very—unless—that is, you are a person who cares about his or her personal well being.

Most people exhibit the "I don't really care" behaviors. That is until "tragedy," sickness or disease sets in. Even then, some people still don't care enough to stop the behaviors, which, as surely as the sun will set, will cause them serious health consequences. This fact is ordained in Nature. No one can violate the laws of life and escape the consequences.

Some Guiding Principles

What if…what if someone really wanted to take charge, to take control of his or her personal health, happiness and disease-free existence? After being armed with good and reliable information—such as might be written by any Natural Hygienist, including this writer—you now need only make one decision and commit to one behavior: (a) ideally, decide to consume only

(FVNS) fruits, vegetables, nuts and seeds—organically grown and uncooked; and (b) make a commitment to implement health producing behaviors into your lifestyle.

Failing to live healthfully will doom anyone to a reduced quality of life, to drugging, cutting, burning, to pain and suffering, unhappiness and to the curtailment of longevity. And this is so, not because Natural Hygienists say so, but because Mother God, the First Cause, the Unmoved Mover, Jehovah, Allah, the Great Spirit, The Creator, has preordained that it be so. And neither vast sums of money nor vibrant youth can suspend these laws of The Creator.

Confusions and Frustrations

When there is motivation to change, individuals tend to become even more dependent; they begin to ask questions, but often will not make important decisions unless they are given believable answers. And, almost anyone "of authority," can come across as being 'believable.' Conflicting information and sometimes-painful errors often fling individuals into outrageous fear or, at least, waning resolve to effect significant behavioral changes in their consumptive lifestyles.

What happens, simply, is that people become stampeded, either by their own erroneous actions or by misinformation from "believable" sources. Beware of so-called 'celebrity endorsers.' Ever wonder how Magic Johnson "knew" he "had" 'the A.I.D.S. virus?' Especially when it never has been established that 'HIV' causes anything and 'tests' for HIV have been "a fraud from day one?" Magic Johnson's wife later thanked God for her husband's "miraculous cure." Magic Johnson changed behaviors, backing off twenty-five years of drugging (for athletic pain, injury and whatever!).

The options about which we spoke earlier still may be exercised: one can arm herself or himself with 'reliable information.' And, one can commit herself or himself to implementing fundamental changes in his or her consumptive lifestyle. These changes, incidentally, are discoverable in the literature of Natural Hygiene [Contacts: Dr. Bernard Jensen Retreat, Route 1, Box 52, Escondido, CA 92025; Organic Wellness Crusade, PO Box 7219, Beverly Hills, CA 90212-7219, and Dr. V. V. Vetrano at The Rest of Your Life Health Retreat, PO Box 102, Barksdale, TX 78828].

There are no big mysteries: no complicated systems and rules; no perplexing terms and technical language; no difficult-to-perform or illogical activities. The Natural Hygiene system is easy to understand, and it meets the 'common sense test.' Its dictum is: "Eat your foods mostly raw; eat only what you like raw; and appropriately meet your other needs of life." 'Proof' or evidence will be the wonderful and observable changes in your life within days of adapting hygienic behaviors.

To those who know, but do not tell the truth, Dr. Bernard Jensen declares: *"We are committing a crime when we do not let people know that they are doing a serious wrong to themselves if they do not live a clean, healthful life insofar as it is possible in our civilized world of today. Failure to teach the public that they are producing bad tissue because of bad living habits, and keeping them from knowing that they are producing the soil for a possible cancerous growth as the result—should be considered a crime. Public education on the correct way to live has been neglected far beyond what it should be, and one of these days we will recognize this as our greatest need."*

Ihre Gesundheit, (Germany), by this writer, variously published in four countries as **A *Guide to Healthy Living*** (Nigeria) **The *American Diet*** (Japan), first appeared in 1986 (Publius Publishers, Pacific Palisades, CA) as ***Helping Hand: 8-Day Diet Programs for People Who Care about Wellness***. The book is becoming a classic guidebook for initiating and managing a healthful living lifestyle.

The Shelton Library, John Robbins' ***Diet for a New America,*** and other books are readily available.

The Road to Great Wealth

Traveling the only 'road' to sickness and disease-free living leads one straight to organic, uncooked fruits, vegetables, nuts and seeds. The road involves exercise, natural light and sunshine, and fresh air and positive thinking. But, it also encompasses sufficient rest and peaceful sleep; warm surroundings and friendly faces; quiet shelter and safe places. You must be often surrounded by individuals who have sworn off consumption of animal foods. You must often see and talk with people who are committed to maximum control over their own destinies, and who have concerns for the environment.

On this great road to a disease-free existence, one would have to have left behind milk consumption; caffeine from coffee, tea and soft drinks; processed foods ("as seen on TV"); desserts and snack foods; ice cream and yogurts; beer, wine and spirits; tobacco products; animal products; condiments, such as salt, pepper and salad dressings; and everything that (a) ever was capable of independent movement, (b) has been tampered with or enriched, (c) does not grow in natural earth, and/or (d) has not reached your consumption table without detrimental interference by "middle men."

Remember that simple truth we talked about earlier? That absolute principle upon which any and all disease free existence must depend? As Spike Lee, the moviemaker put it, "Doing the right thing" by your body also delivers important benefits to your mind; important enhancement of your spirit; and an increased level of happiness and quality of life. You should try it…for about five or six years; you'll never go back to eating animal flesh, or to drinking 'soft drinks' or alcohol! And, it would have been years since you put so-called medications into your body. By that time, you long ago would have given up consuming refined sugar, and all its variations, such as breads, donuts, cakes, cookies, chocolates (candies in general), pies and other starches.

Eating mostly organically grown fruits, vegetables, nuts and seeds—uncooked; drinking only purified or distilled water, and the juices of 'frugetables' (the juices of fruits and vegetables: Anderson, 1992), all in combinations that respect the metabolic requirements of the body: these will lead to vibrant health, energetic wellness, happy disposition, enhanced quality of life and meaningful longevity.

In the words of Dr. T. C. Fry, "Disease is an extraordinary body effort to eliminate encumbering morbid matters that impede its normal function. The body initiates the emergency and preempts its energies to redirect the detoxification and healing. When the body has accomplished its objectives, we are said to be well which, indeed, we are. The body, in its great wisdom, has restored us to wellness."

Chapter Four

Alternatives to Dying Prematurely

Individuals die, not from disease as it is commonly believed, but from cause. 'Something' causes this organism to malfunction, 'abort life' or die prematurely, which if otherwise nourished and left alone would function fine and thrive. Such a simple fact 'escapes' conscious recognition because of our 'civilized training' [cultural education from pre-birth to around age 13, the period during which most of our 'important learning' takes place]. Education has been defined as "the process of teaching children the values and culture of their parents and elders." Certain other learnings are said to be 'common sense.' Children know of 'traumatic' deaths, which occur long before age 20; but they have little or no knowledge of persons dying of 'natural cause' at age 120 and beyond.

Not only has the relationship between 'diet and early death' not been taught to our children, parents haven't learned it themselves! Studies and practices of Seventh Day Adventists demonstrated earlier in American history a 'causal' relationship between types and quality of food consumed and types and intensities of disease conditions later in life. In recent years, Prof. T. Colin Campbell's, *"The China Study,"* demonstrated anew the absolute connection between quality and character of foods consumed and the incidences of well known 'Western diseases.' Put, simply, according to some studies, "Premature dying, most often, is a result of 'dietary deficiencies!'" The SAD is a primary factor in disease and early death in Western Society, and to an increasing degree in other societies that emulate the West!

In dramatic terms, if one fell from an airplane, the general expectation is that the person would die. If shot in the heart, immediate death would be expected; and if too badly burned, the organism dies. These 'truths' are said to be self-evident. No one argues with these conclusions. These incidents are illustrations of the workings of Natural Law, the law of 'Effects of Cause.' And despite the rare 'chance' one can fall from an airplane and not die, or be shot through the heart and survive, or be seriously burned and overcome—and we have no problem 'allowing for' these exceptions—we reasonably expect death to result.

From our earliest upbringing, we have been taught certain workings of the natural law of "cause and effect." We know, for instance, that little boys drown who fail to swim in deep water. We learn that little girls often die when struck by hit-and-run vehicles. It is during childhood that we learn people get sick and sometimes die [presumably from 'the sickness'].

But, we 'learn' much more about 'cause and effect.' We learn what actions bring us rewards and which actions bring about scorn [or 'spankings!']. Through prenatal 'learning' to the onset of teen years, most of what we learn will form the foundation of our 'inner sanctum' which will govern our behavior and belief structure for the rest of our lives. Once learned, never will we outgrow the notion that "black cats are bad luck!" No matter how many university degrees we earn, or how many humanitarian awards we receive, once learned in childhood, we continue to believe "13 is an evil number, with connections to the devil."

Yet, in our wisdom and in our acknowledgments, we have overlooked something very simple, but extremely important: we can see the fall from an airplane [the 'cause'] leading to death [the 'effect']; but, our 'intelligence' [civilized training and upbringing'] does not permit us "to see" <u>causes</u> of less dramatic dying, or of 'slow death.' It is almost as if our consciousness has been programmed to see 'death by cause' only if it is sudden, as in dying "by the electric chair!" or "killed in an auto accident." Our minds 'permit' millions to die from 'a virus,' without ever confirming the meaning and true characteristics of ***virus.***

Nor does our upbringing permit us to rationalize or analyze our predicament. We are not even permitted, in civilized society, "to know" 'the cause' of death. Why a body dies can be declared only by 'a licensed physician;' otherwise, 'the cause of death' might remain 'unofficial.' But, what is the point of all of this, anyway? Just this, really: you and I are not credited, in our society, with the intelligence to <u>know why people die</u>. Therefore, there is no credibility given to either our possibility of knowing or to our <u>need to know</u> *what is actually killing us*.

When we think of beloved relatives, or friends for that matter, who have recently died, we tend "to think" of the 'official reasons' given us, why they are no longer alive. Even in cases where we knew differently—and believed differently—we tend "to accept" the 'official cause of death' as we have been told. The point being made here is not that one might have died of self-inflicted wounds while the 'certificate of death' reads "Complications of congestive coronary disease." But, rather that one dies from alcohol consumption and the certificate reads 'liver failure.'

The <u>cause</u> is alcohol consumption; the <u>effect</u> is [premature] death. By having the 'cause' excluded from our mental process [which is what happens when we accept the 'liver failure' explanation]. We 'forget' the death was <u>premature</u>, or unnecessary [at the time it occurred]. So, while there is no escaping death—for any of us—there is merit in not advancing the hour of death prematurely. But, because we do not 'know' <u>what causes death</u>, it seems to 'surprise' us when someone dies—other than 'accident victims,' old people and military personnel, of course.

Yet sixty people are killed every year in hospitals for one killed during 10 years of war in Vietnam! The hospital deaths are all caused by "physician mal-practice." And there is no public outrage! Why? The media 'told' the public of the 5,000+ who were killed each year in Vietnam, but do not tell of the 300,000+ who "are killed yearly in hospitals."

When we do not know 'the cause' of premature death, we cannot know (1) that medications cause death, (2) that so-called 'recreational' drugs cause death, (3) that chemicals cause death, (4) that starvation causes death, (5) that polluted water and polluted air cause death, (6) that beer and wine cause death, (7) that tobacco products cause death, (8) that over medicated animal and flesh foods cause death, (9) that cooked, denatured foods and condiments cause death, and finally, (10) that there in precious little death without a traceable dietary cause. And, *never is the cause of death 'disease.'* Disease is only the manifestation' or symptom [pre-effect] of the premature death [effect] which follows 'the natural order of events.'

Three Causes of Death

Since we have established the self-evident fact that death must have a cause, which we—despite our upbringing—can know, we can examine "all causes of death" and find but three: (1) death caused by insufficient nutrients or Natural Law; (2) death caused by 'fatal imposition' or trauma; and (3) death caused by the 'retained effects' of "stuff" housed too long in the organism (body and mind storage)!

Let us examine these 'three causes of death' more carefully. Natural Law is operative when, from no 'causal action' related to the organism, it is imperfectly created and malfunctions so severely as to short-circuit its existence, and dies prematurely. Or, when "the life cycle is complete" for that individual; or it is fatally impacted by lightning or other natural phenomena. "If we accept the proposition that more than 90% of premature deaths result from 'dietary causes' or "nutrient deficiencies," then it follows that this construct, indeed, falls under the purview of Natural Law.

By contrast, 'fatal imposition' or trauma covers a multitude of observable causes of death. All accidents—though 'caused' by something or someone—must be considered either sudden or subtle imposition on the organism, and are either immediately fatal or fatal over a longer period. "Recreational drug use," according to Professor Peter Duesberg, molecular biologist at the University of California, Berkeley, "is the direct cause of so-called A.I.D.S." If Dr. Duesberg is correct—and this writer believes he is—then A.I.D.S. [describes] what will or is likely to happen to an organism from the 'stuff' consumed by that organism.

The third cause of death, then, is precisely that death is precipitated by the actions of 'toxic stuff,' too much and too long housed inside the organism. Refer to what you 'know' [have been led to believe] about A.I.D.S., for example. Do you know of anyone over forty years old who has died "of the disease" [except, of course, those "high profile" individuals like Rock Hudson, who were instrumental in 'catching the media's attention!']? Have you known other diseases which are "interested" only in persons in the 45-age range? And when you count back, say 25-30 years, how old was the person 25 years before death occurred? What do you 'know' or can surmise about the social or wellness lifestyle of that younger person?

Of course this line of questioning is 'not popular.' Nor is it intended to be. The point here is rather simple, really. Despite the fact that 'toxic substances' housed within the organism will, eventually and often, lead to death, such death is seldom so rapid as to put the occurrence in the category of 'trauma or fatal imposition" [which carries a more timely implication]. So, the conclusion of Professor Peter Duesberg, Ph.D. is consistent with our own analysis. The subtle dynamic here is that when *cause* precedes *effect* by 5, 10, 15, 20 or 25 years, we tend to **not** see the connection; and, we are helped in our 'blindness' by those whose purposes are best served.

Ultimately from ignorance [the mis-teachings in our culture], we bring about premature death more slowly or more rapidly—depending upon our actions <u>and beliefs</u>. One whose lifestyle consumes ice cream is likely to outlive one whose lifestyle consumes cocaine. People who use salt (and pepper) on their food are more likely to come down with high blood pressure or hypertension [reported on death certificates as 'the cause' of death] than those who squeeze on a few drops of lemon juice. Clearly, what causes ultimate death are the nutrient-deficient substances ["seasonings"] which disrupt normal body functioning and ultimately lead to the demise of one or more body functions or organs.

Some people have died of so-called A.I.D.S., no doubt, who did not have even a 'common cold.' Such deaths occur when belief structures are so contaminated with 'false information' that it results in 'programming' the organisms' mental mechanisms. This results in the production and over-production of chemicals, both in the brain and in the rest of the organism, such that these become liabilities. Stored internal chemicals [whether produced by the body or by a manufacturer] exact their toll, and often lead the organism to premature demise. One can—and often does—'will oneself to die.' It is an all too-frequent occurrence. A friend of mine, Dr. Charleston J. Young, once told me about two hobo men during a Chicago winter. They climbed into a boxcar with a 56-degree temperature. One man said to the other, "This is too cold; I just soon die." And, within minutes of his pronouncement, he was dead. What happens in the case of AIDS is that a body that is already nutrient-deprived now tries to cope with the onrush of "recreational chemicals." These exacerbate the crisis and the system simply "shuts down," or in computer terms, "crashes." "First, pathological degeneration occurs; then death follows. The MD tends to see only degeneration. We now see the causes!" Dr. Vetrano assures us.

Search for Another 'Cause of Death'

The real "tragedy" of the AIDS epidemic is the 'gross denial' associated with it. *People not only rationalize that drug usage causes AIDS, but they tend to 'glorify' the 'victims' and martyr the dead!* The message this sends in that if you kill yourself using drugs, one day people will walk and raise funds in your memory! Eventually, "They will discover 'a cure' for our not killing ourselves taking drugs!" Dr. Young admitted in a moment of levity.

Lest we engage 'oversimplification,' let us pursue other possible 'causes' of death. What of the "disease notion" of death? Have we sufficiently examined it? To the extent that even the medical establishment confirms that "disease symptoms" refer to 'indications or evidence of organic disease,' we say, again: disease is not a 'cause' of death, but could be a description of the 'shape and form' of the onset of death. To see the 'cause' of the eventual death, attention must be turned, back to some earlier action—direct or vicarious—timely or long term. And, so far such action results from (1) nutrient deficiency (natural phenomena) (2) trauma or (3) body storage. Dr. Vetrano adds, "These cause the organic changes that finally end in death."

"Heart disease kills more Americans than any other single cause!" you might read, from time to time, in the world's most prestigious newspapers. However, such a statement is a complete falsehood. 'Heart disease' is but "a description" of how death was prematurely activated. What causes the deterioration in the arteries or the vessels in the heart, or what 'fatally impacted' its vital functioning might have been weakened muscles due to the over consumption of caffeine or from the lack of sufficient exercise. The heart 'failed,' but from nutrient deprivation and related handicaps.

Natural Hygiene [that system of biology researched by Herbert M. Shelton, N.D., et.al.], abounds with 'scientific evidence,' for example, that only in countries where citizens consume animal and flesh products [pork, beef, seafood, fowl] is there notable incidents of premature death from "heart disease." Japan, for example, a country which prior to its 'Westernized diet had very little heart disease is beginning to show serious heart disease statistics. Additional evidence points to alcohol consumption, drug usage, coffee-tea-soft drink, and to what some refer to as "stress" [synergistic effects of body chemicals, a liability], and also from tobacco usage.

So far, however, we have not found 'another cause' of death. Since 'heart disease' is only the "symptom," we have to look farther for the 'cause.' Once the cause is found, we know immediately that sickness or death resulted from either (a) natural law, (b) trauma, or (c) body storage. As yet, no other 'causal factor' has surfaced.

But what about genetic, degenerative and communicable diseases? Are these not other causes of death? If we are to be consistent, the obvious answer is "No." We have demonstrated by various examples that disease or "dis-ease" is 'a description,' not a 'cause.' Genetic or degenerative or 'communicable' all describe "disease," which is the subject or noun: and we have shown it to be not the cause.

'Communicable Disease' or 'Contagion'

Earlier we discussed how we were raised to accept certain things as being 'true,' whether they were or not. Classic examples are (1) Santa Clause comes; he brings toys; he comes 'down the chimney.' (2) The 'Tooth Fairy' pulls our tooth; or takes it from our mouths or pillows; and exchanges the tooth for a coin or present. (3) 'The Stork' delivers Mommy's baby [Dad had nothing to do with it!]. Whether these are 'innocent' beliefs or not is hardly the issue. Fact of the matter is that we are taught early, thoroughly and continuously, how to have 'the taught mind' say "yes" to what the 'untaught mind' would utter "no" to.

The significance of this point is twofold: 1) If one can 'catch' a 'disease' [which is itself, but 'a description,' remember?], there is no need to ever 'know' the cause of any subsequent, premature sickness, suffering or premature death. And, 2) since we have been taught to 'believe and accept' that "fat Santa" can come down a house chimney, what is wrong with believing and accepting that we can "catch" 'a description!' Surely, one makes as much 'sense' as does the other.

In Christianity we are taught (1) Jesus was born of a virgin, without assistance from Joseph [or any other male]; (2) Three days after his death, "Jesus rose from the dead;" (3) Jesus was 'The Only Begotten Son' of God, 'The Father' ["a Spirit"]; (4) Jesus "came down from Heaven;" and (5) "Was sacrificed [executed] for our sins."

Children grow up; and their beliefs 'grow up' with them. Now, as adults, we continue to believe the same 'illogical stuff' which was "okay for children to be taught," because that is how 'our culture' is transmitted from one generation to another. And so, the stage is set...for the balance of most lives. The pattern is similar for 'truth' not taught.

But, the stakes get bigger and better. What if you are trained in allopathic [conventional] medicine and I am trained in theology [Christianity]? You and your colleagues need 'mysticism' and "unreality" to sustain your exalted 'connection' to life and death, just as do my associates and I. So we 'allow' you the *'theory of contagion'* to sustain your profession, and you 'allow us the doctrine of the *'resurrection of Jesus'* to sustain ours. As a result, we both continue to benefit from how our children [now adults] 'think, behave, and believe.' No harm done: we have not 'hurt' anyone. What is more, we have taken vows to only 'do good.' So, "The man *caught* syphilis, before he died and received life everlasting [*was saved*] by the power of the risen Jesus!"

This is not intended as either a refutation of religion [Christianity] or of a repudiation of any fundamental 'doctrine' of conventional medicine. Instead, we want to show only that what we believe affects what is, or can be, 'real' for us. And generally speaking if one thing 'satisfies' us as being true, there is little need to anticipate any other 'truth.' In other words, once we accept the notion that we "can catch" a fatal disease [description of a body dying], there is little need to look farther for causes. There is no need to remember that essential minerals are absent from our soils, that animals are filled with drugs, and that plant life is laden with pesticides and radiation. In reading this manuscript, Dr. Vetrano was moved to remark, "Dr. Anderson, you have a new—unique—way of making people see the real causes of death. This book is a real eye opener!"

Let us test our theory against the backdrop of all the death and dying that occurred in Africa and Europe [Ethiopia not long ago and the former Soviet Union more recently.] We are told that these people have died and are dying "from war, starvation, and disease." Now, we already know, despite what we elect to believe, ***that any disease is but a description,*** not a cause of death. But, what of 'starvation?' What of 'war?' Is starvation a description or a 'cause?' In a sense, it is neither; it is more an 'effect.' Fail to provide sufficient nutrients for the body and it will starve…to death!

And even when 'starvation' or 'war is an effect, it 'describes' what happened [prior to dying], but it still does not refer us back to 'the cause' [lack of nutrients or violent trauma]. By accepting the public explanation that these souls are dying "from starvation or from war," are we given not one but two 'causes' of death in Europe and other parts of the world? That is the question. Now, for the 'Santa Clause answer' [referred to in this way because we have already demonstrated our ability to accept 'unreality' by learned behavior from our youth]. This skill helps us to categorize 'information' for storing or for ignoring. Remember, the "25 law enforcement officers did not violate Rodney King's constitutional rights; it only appeared that way on television! They were in fear of their lives (from this lone, unarmed black man!)!"

What if Attorney Larry Shulman and Dick Gregory were correct [WOL-AM Radio, Washington, D.C., December 31, 1992, 9 AM]? What if the people of Somalia [East Africa] were showing 'the evidence' [disease symptoms] which result when toxic chemicals and/or nuclear waste products are disposed of in the midst of populated areas within those countries? What if such pollution undermined crop growing?

What if it poisoned water supplies? What if in exchange for the privilege to dump, "food and drugs [medication]" were promised, in addition to millions of dollars? Can you see how raising such questions as these help point our way toward real 'causes' of the deaths which occurred? Guess what? If Shulman and Gregory were correct about Somalia, what of other African, Asian, and Island nations where corrupt and misinformed leaders have been co-opted by the misinformation and self-interest of the West in general and of the United States in particular? What country or countries will be next? Dare we take another look at "AIDS in Africa?"

Getting back to the three causes of death, certainly starvation comes under the banner of 'trauma.' Since, during starvation, the body lacks substance, it certainly is not being diminished by 'stuff stored' within. Rather, it is traumatized by neglect, <u>by the political violence of 'hunger</u>.' Dying without any 'defense' mechanisms, the press incorrectly reports various 'disease conditions' [descriptions of dying, complications of pre-dying, and rather certain estimations of pending deaths].

To Whom Do You Belong?

The principle is the same, whether or not we can see the 'cause of death' among relatives and friends, or among Africans, Europeans, or Asians. One thing is certain: <u>there can be no constructive solution for a problem until it is, first, perceived</u>. In other words, until we are able to understand our upbringing it is hard for us to realize how 'ignorant' we are. The best-kept secrets in society are totally exposed right before our eyes [which we have been systematically trained 'how' to 'see' and 'how to <u>not</u> see'].

When it comes right down to it, the question each of us must ask is: To whom do I [my body, mind, soul, and spirit] belong? Does society own me? Do I belong to my religion? Am I subject only to the whims of the state? Do I belong to 'special interest groups [the meat industry, alcohol and beverages, dairy, fish, poultry, medical, pharmaceutical, advertisement, political, etc., etc., etc.] or do I belong to myself? Or do I belong to my God?

If I belong to myself, I want to know what causes me to malfunction, and potentially die prematurely. In my state of higher spiritual awareness, I am also concerned about what causes the premature deaths of millions of my fellow humans. Once I know that tobacco products will bring about premature death, the imposition of cigarettes in my life becomes 'criminal' no matter from whom the imposition comes.

If I am content to die—less prematurely—from 'natural causes,' I am compelled to learn what actions contribute to a significant reduction in my 'normal' life cycle. In other words, according to the science of Natural Hygiene, much of what we consume in the name of food and beverage [except organically grown, raw fruits, vegetable, nuts and seeds] contributes to our demise—some things more rapidly than others. Milk is going to do me more harm than will orange juice; sugar more than wheat; nuclear waste more than residential garbage.

My actions must become deliberate. I must source out and validate reliable information. ***I must religiously avoid as many of the known impediments to good health as I can control.*** And I must look beyond my immediate environment, into the larger community, even into the community of nations; and I must show my 'righteous indignation' concerning acts that are 'criminal,' whether against an Indonesian Islander or against my friend Joe, down the street, or indeed against by very own organism.

"Life Cycle"

The concept, "life cycle," is a 'mystical' notion which could involve any aberration, from 'ancient ancestors' to a prior existence, to a presupposed 'pending state' [being resurrected or transcending this plain]. This line of thinking and believing differs from what we will demonstrate as the cycle of life. However, before getting more into this part of our discussion, it is necessary to clarify one more aspect of 'the theory of disease.'

The Merck Manual [the bible of the medical profession] does not list 'disease' in its index; therefore, no page references are given, and no 'definition.' This, despite the fact that we are urged in the Foreword to Edition 15 to "...check the Index whenever you require information, even on unusual subjects or those not commonly found in other texts" [earlier Merck Manuals?]. Yet in the "Foreword to Volumes I and II" by Robert Berkow, M.D. we are told: "Furthermore, disease discussions include relevant data about incidence, epidemiology, etiology, pathophysiology, symptoms and signs and laboratory data, as well as differential diagnosis and treatment."

If you cannot "see" 'Santa Claus' in the previous statement note that the first 196 pages of ***The Merck Manual*** [Published by Merck Sharp & Dohme Research Laboratories, Division of Merck & Co., Inc. (drug manufacturers!)] are concerned with "Infectious and Parasitic Diseases." The entire manual is over 1700 pages, all about 'diseases,' a subject too 'unimportant' to be defined, despite the fact the book is distributed to medical practitioners worldwide [and they use it as their "bible" in practicing their allopathic profession!]. Page one gives us a hint, *"A healthy individual lives in harmony with his normal body flora but this balance may be disturbed by disease."*

Yet hopeful, we pursue our quest "for information." And, under "Respiratory Viral Diseases," on page 121, we are told, "Viral infections of the respiratory tract are acute illnesses with local and systemic manifestations." Finally, on page 193, with the admission of "Diseases of Uncertain Etiology," we are advised, that 'Sarcoidosis' is "a multisystem granulomatous disorder of unknown etiology, characterized histologically by epithelioid tubercles involving various organs or tissues with symptoms dependent on the site and degree of involvement."

John H. Tilden, M.D., a physician for 67 years, sought to swim upstream of his profession and resolve the 'great mystery' by identifying "disease." His conclusion is found in his book entitled, ***Toxemia: The Basic Cause of Disease***. "In the process of tissue building—metabolism—there is cell building—anabolism—and cell destruction—catabolism. The broken down tissue is toxic and in health when nerve energy is normal, it is eliminated from the blood as fast as evolved. When nerve energy is dissipated from any cause, physical, mental or bad habits the body becomes *enervated* [emphasis this author's]. When enervated, elimination is checked; causing a retention of toxins within the blood tissues which we name toxemia."

Let's look at where we are: We find no 'definition' of disease in the 'bible' of the medical profession, but references to (1) diseases as manifestation, (2) diseases as symptoms, (3) disease as related to 'the site and degree of involvement' in the body, and finally, (4) Dr. Tilden who offers a detailed description of the cause of the description, namely poison build-up internally or by trauma. Therefore, it appears consistent that while 'disease' points us toward the 'effect' in Natural Law, Dr. Tilden's 'toxemia' points us toward the 'cause' as the universal principle by which all Creation is governed. ***In short, the 'purpose' of disease (process) is restoration of wellness.***

The publisher said that my book, ***Helping Hand: 8-Day Diet Programs for People Who Care About Wellness*** (Publius, 1986) was "right on the mark" and that book referenced a report in the ***New England Journal of Medicine*** which affirmed that, "After thirty years, the war on cancer had been lost," and the general public was being urged to "look more toward prevention rather than to cures." Prevention amounts to not causing disease, and is predicated upon proper consumption and adequate elimination, both physically and mentally.

Chapter Five

Understanding Cancers

Oncology literature, generally made available to grieving individuals and their families, tells us there are more than 100 different disease conditions diagnosed and treated as "cancer." The plethora of medical tests confirming analyses and treatment modalities is correlated to "evidence of metastasis," or the spreading of identical tumor tissues. My description of 'cancer tissue' is ***rotting human flesh!***

A million people are diagnosed with "cancer" annually in America, and the medical establishment realizes an average of $100,000 per person, or about 10% of its annual income, second only to income from performing "tests and examinations."

Despite the above, 9 out of 10 people diagnosed with cancer "do not, in fact, have cancer but tumors," which a non-enervated body routinely eliminates during a two-to-five week 'therapeutic fast.' Some recognized names of oncology's "more than 100 cancers" are: Hodgkin's disease, Leukemia, Colon Carcinoma, Primary Malignant Metastatic Lesions of Bone, and various connective tissue disorders might be variously referred to and/or diagnosed as "cancer."

Others are self-identifying, such as breast cancer, skin cancer, cancer of the colon and rectum (Adenocarcinomas), throat cancer, prostate cancer, liver cancer, stomach cancer, Primary Lung Carcinoma (lung cancer), and many others.

Crisis of Toxemia

Herbert M. Shelton, N.D., Ph.D., John H. Tilden, M.D., Alvenia M. Fulton, N.D., Ph.D., the late "Queen Mother of Wholistic Science," and others agree the above symptoms and conditions each describes ***a crisis of toxemia***, internally, externally, and/or both. This "wholistic view" of *effect* correspondingly favors unconventional theories. But, conventional medicine takes a different view.

Recommended procedures depend upon where the tumor appears in the body, and on how much metastasis is evident. ***Surgery, radiation and chemotherapy*** are the most recommended treatments. Other drugs—sometimes called 'miracle drugs' or experimental drugs—support the general notion in conventional medicine that "We have no cure for cancer."

This declaration is made—usually soon after the diagnosis—so that the "patient is not given false hope." Instead, the promise is to "do everything we can to make the patient comfortable and not experience unbearable pain (for what time he or she has left)." ***The psychological effects are, perhaps, more devastating*** than "giving false hope." A UCLA study shows some ninety percent of people given the "fatal cancer diagnosis" die, not from their disease conditions, but from mental devastation!

Systemic Poisoning

Look, again, at the above scenarios: First, not all 100 different manifestations are understood to be evidence of systemic poisoning. Dietary poisoning is only partially acknowledged by allopathic or the conventional medical community. Surely, as Natural Hygiene holds, these 100-plus manifestations consistently express the body's innate efforts to rid itself of un-eliminated poisons.

Failing to be eliminated, these poisons are cumulative—and life threatening. Locations in the body where tissues show 'abnormal growth' patterns, or fail to generate 'normal new cell growth' could be understood or likened to that part of a potato which rots. 'Rotting' human flesh is a concept found neither in medical literature—nor, for that matter, in hygienic literature either.

A Rotting Potato

Allopathic procedures resemble what one might do who wanted to 'prolong the potential' of a rotting potato: Either (1) cut out the rot, hoping to "get all of it," (2) apply radiation, or (3) treat the potato with drugs or chemicals (chemotherapy).

All these procedures are fatalistic. They deal neither with removing the causal factors nor with reducing the cumulative poisoning. For the potato—in the latter phase of its life cycle—such pessimism might be justified. But, the human organism is dynamic; it is alive and ever changing.

Unlike the rotting potato—whose message is not one of cumulative toxemia but an indication of the end of a life cycle—human tissues die and are eliminated, and there is rebirth continuously. But, if not eliminated from the body, these dead and dying tissues become deadly poisons and will 'kill' the entire organism. "Remember," reminds Dr. Vetrano, "our immune cells—phagocytes—eat up the delirious cells." Thus, when immune or white cells are too few, toxicity builds up and death is more likely to occur. Drugs and chemical poisons kill off white blood cells.

Dr. T. C. Fry describes cancer as an "endpoint in a pathological progression arising from pathogenic substances and influences. In reality, cancer begins with the first transgression of our biological disposition visited upon us by innocent and unaware parents." All of us, therefore, are 'carriers of cancer' and when, or if, we will experience a "cancer crisis" one day, it is a matter of lifestyle, time and accumulation.

Beginnings of 'Cancer' In Mother or Child

Natural Hygiene is consistent with the position that disease begins when the infant body is filled with substances biologically unsuited to its inherited faculties and physiological capabilities. Dr. Fry concurs when he says, "Even mother's milk, the best food of all for an infant, is pathogenic if the mother eats an atrocious diet or indulges drugs of any kind including coffee, alcohol, tobacco, teas, and chocolates which, unfortunately, most American nursing women do." He concludes, "This and other poor practices foisted upon the child begets a long train of pathology that culminates in cancer—for both the mother and the offspring."

In foreign societies, perhaps, major culprits are impure drinking water, toxic waste, chemicals, polluted air, and compromised food quality. The net results, however, are the same as in the West.

Ingestion of coffee, tea, soft drinks, candies, cookies, birthday cakes, alcohol, vinegar, medicines, cooked foods such as pizza, meats, greasy chips, and 'snack foods' build up into a cesspool of intestinal toxicosis. This plus the body's own discarded wastes are either eliminated or they, too, become carcinogens or deadly poison that threaten the survival of individual cells.

Dr. Fry describes how the body responds to such conditions: "In protecting itself from toxic substances, the body creates cysts, sacs, polyps, wens, and tumors around the morbid materials (carcinogens) for the purpose of encapsulating and quarantining them from the body's vital tissues and organs."

Free Radicals or Aberrant Cells

We agree, carcinogens cause 'cancer.' When toxins saturate the body, as we have been discussing, the impact threatens the integrity and life of cells. When facing death from deprivation of oxygen or intoxication with deadly substances, an organized cell of body economy may secede from the tissue (the body union) and lead an independent existence. The body's faculties endeavor to eliminate the aberrant cells and, with vitality, these innate faculties usually succeed.

Cells that secede may be malignant (that is, they may reproduce by mitosis or division). What happens, as Dr. Fry agrees, is the body is not able to quarantine or imprison the independent cells, hence they may travel (metastasize) or arise in entirely new locations. Pretty much like foam atop a running stream or rot in a potato. All that 'stuff' (described as "aberrant cells," "free radicals," "tumors" or whatever) is nothing more or less than "floating waste material." Left unchecked (***uneliminated***), it will poison an organ or the entire system, and "death from cancer" results. ***The 'remedy,' at this stage is detoxification (through therapeutic fasting and rest); while, pure remedy (earlier on) is prevention.*** My friend, Dr. Harvey Diamond (co-author of ***Fit for Life***) has demonstrated in a new book that "you can overcome cancer!"

Herbert M. Sheldon, N.D., Vivian Virginia Vetrano, M.D. and others agree with T.C. Fry that "the chain of disease progression begins with enervation," that condition of the body when nerve energies are so spent as to put the body in a condition it is unable to adequately carry out its eliminative tasks. What is referred to as "the common cold" is, perhaps, the most recognized symptom of the onset of enervation. This is precisely why there never was, and never can be, "a cure for the common cold." Rest and restoration to enhance and insure elimination are 'the cure.'

Retained Toxic Substances

Un-eliminated wastes and toxic substances are retained in the blood and tissues; and this leads to toxicosis, bacterial fermentation and putrefaction. Add consumed toxins to the body's own wastes, when not eliminated it all becomes morbid.

This morbid material gives rise to ***irritation.*** "Irritation manifests as discomforts: itches, rashes, queasy feelings, qualms, and yet other symptoms." When the cause of the irritation is continued, the body will take "emergency rescue action lest it be overwhelmed by the train of toxic materials."

Natural Hygiene writers and researches contend that this emergency or massive eliminative effort on the part of the body is symptomized by *inflammation.* Inflammation is sometimes referred to as fevers or 'itises."

Boils, papillae, and pustules are created, then lesions (which can be external or internal) which are called *ulceration*. Ulcers can occur on the outer skin or the inner skin, in the mucous membranes. "Ulcers or open sores can occur within tissues and within organs as well." **The innate intelligence of the body always takes steps to survive.** *The body heals itself, as long as it has the nerve energy to do so.*

When it is able to sufficiently eliminate ***this deadly toxic saturation***, these ulcers are healed by a process called fibrillation or scarring or granulated tissue formation. When the body cannot eliminate toxic materials, it strives to isolate them from vital functions by forming sacs called cysts, polyps, wens, tumors, etc.

How Tumors Arise

When the body's own innate intelligence 'decides' this morbid material cannot be eliminated, it uses its next best option: it attempts to isolate this poisonous material in the least used areas, as women's breasts and uterine cavities, and in men's prostates, or in sacs elsewhere in the body.

What the medical profession describes as "metastasized disease condition" [or "the spreading of the disease"] is what we describe as the continuation of the 'cycle of poisoning.' That is what all 'cancers' are.

Dr. Fry puts it this way: "When toxic saturation progresses to the point that the existence of cells is threatened, body cells may withdraw from the body context and strive to exist independently, parasitizing upon the parent organism for sustenance. A good example of independent cells is warts. Warts are aberrant cells which the body has exiled to the outside [of the body] but continue to nourish."

How long does the cancer chronology take? How much time does one have to correct an abusive consumptive lifestyle? Perhaps the most disturbing answer to this question is, likewise, offered by Dr. Fry when he tells us: "It is a sad commentary that the primary cause of death among our youth is cancer [emphasis added]. The situation is getting worse inasmuch as only 37% of our young get any exercise at all in school, and 92% cannot pass a minimum fitness test. The average American child/teenager is a 'couch potato' who watches television 6 ½ hours daily and consumes train loads of snack foods, especially grease-laden chips, pizzas, and other carcinogenic fare."

Dynamic Human Organism

Treating the dynamic, human organism as if "cancer" is the end of the human life cycle is totally misunderstanding how the human organism becomes 'diseased' in the first place. Such approaches to 'treatment' bear strong testimony that there is little or no perception that (a) systemic toxemia exists within the organism; (b) 'various manifestations' might appear; (c) when not eliminated, premature death generally results; or that (1) internal toxicity can be reduced when the retained 'stuff' is eliminated; (2) behaviors which brought on the crises are changed to wellness regiments; and (3) the body's own innate healing powers are understood, respected and assisted—primarily by limited interference.

The big difference between the rotting potato and 'rotting' within the human organism is that the potato has no capacity to eliminate what will ultimately lead to its reversion back to nature. ***With sufficient behavior modification, time and nerve energy, the human organism has the innate capacity to cleanse itself, and to change its direction.*** For this reason, "it is never too late to change behaviors!"

Reversing Some 'Cancers'

Some 'cancers' can be reversed in the human organism (1) if the organism wills it so; (2) if there have not been organ failures; (3) if the individual has access to reliable information; (4) if behavior is changed such that poisoning of the organism is reduced to a minimum; and (5) if the level of retained toxins is significantly reduced, primarily through the body's own eliminative processes.

Changing Behaviors and Beliefs

None of the above can occur without fundamental changes in the behaviors which are inconsistent with the principles espoused in Natural Hygiene and confirmed by a wellness lifestyle (Visit the Web Site: http://www.organicwellness.com).

A fundamental beginning is supported in this volume. Because humans are creatures of habit—some of which are addictive habits—any lay person is likely to require knowledgeable and abundant support through the transition to restored well being.

There was a time in America, for example, when people died "of natural causes." In today's market economy, natural death has little monetary value; so, people die of "cancer!" And they die of AIDS. Both of these 'impostors' reflect the same dynamics: the storage of poisons, which are not eliminated, causing cellular derangement, leading to the demise of those individuals. They also illustrate how the medical establishment merchandizes "death and dying" (largely at the expense of the general public, as taxpayers are saddled with paying their bills).

"Individuals who get diagnoses of cancer and shun medical treatment survive an average of 12 ½ years. Those who submit to medical treatment live an average of only three years. This is remarkable inasmuch as over 90% of those who are diagnosed with cancer do not, in fact, have cancer! This testifies to the deadliness of radiation, surgery, and chemotherapy." (UCLA study, 1986)

Cancer is a well-entrenched medical industry. The American population is the primary marketplace, and it is controlled by the world's super rich who are primarily British. Cancer is, unfortunately, one of the primary weapons in the medical arsenal for perpetrating death upon those whom the super rich call 'useless eaters' and consumers of the world's precious resources, which they regard as theirs. Incidentally, the [medical] system strips most cancer sufferers of their accumulated worldly possessions before they are 'permitted' to die.

'Cancer' As 'Big Business'

In 1971, says Dr. Fry, the United States Congress voted $1 billion dollars for cancer research. 24 years later that allocation was $24 billion. In 1971, 350,000 deaths were attributed to cancer; today (1995), 550,000 deaths a year are attributed to cancer. You might say, "That is not an alarming increase, given 24 years." You are correct. But, remember this: cancer now has to share its deaths with so-called A.I.D.S. Each cancer or AIDS patient represents a minimum of $100,000.00 of income for the medical establishment. When allocations for "research" are added, **the cost of death and dying** if known by the general public would be a staggering revelation! According to the principles of Natural Hygiene, much of this wasted cost could be avoided by telling people the truth so that they can make responsible choices.

Now, look what is happening in Africa! A.I.D.S., the new weapon of destruction has been put to work: rid the earth of these masses of people "who are not needed" [and take homosexuals with them, along with many who use 'recreational drugs'. What is it these poor souls have to be striped of? Africa has land, rich land! And those lands are being snatched...as Africans are being poisoned. Africa is useful, too, as a patsy.

According to T.C. Fry, "at the top of the causes of cancer must be listed cooked foods. Cooked foods are deranged foods and the body may suffer many years of extraordinary eliminative crises called colds, flu, 'itises,' upset stomach and flatulence before it looses the vitality to cope. The toxic materials behind these maladies are partially generated by cooking processes, but most are created from the resulting intestinal fermentation and putrefaction."

Fasting and Combating Cancer

Obviously, the best 'cure' for cancer is to prevent it in the first place. But, we have shown how ignorance on the part of our parents starts us on the deadly road. Those who survive their youth can do the following:

1. Locate, read, digest and implement reliable information into consumptive behaviors.
2. Stop indulging those foods and actions that lead to the build up of carcinogens in the intestinal tract.
3. Respect the body's own innate healing intelligence by not interfering with its efforts to carry out its eliminative tasks; and, finally,
4. Incorporate into your lifestyle behaviors which include consumption of raw foods, sunshine and fresh air, exercise, and peaceful surroundings, spiritual tranquility, positive mental attitude, personal warmth, adequate rest and sleep, the affection of kindred spirits, and regular therapeutic fasting. (Anderson, 1992).

It is generally agreed in Natural Hygiene that under the condition of a fast, the body will usually self-digest (utilize) tumors slowly, eliminate the toxic materials and aberrant cells within. Fasting affords the body its full powers and energies in dealing with toxic materials, growths and making of needed repairs.

Fasting from two to five weeks is generally enough time for the body to consume or eliminate a 'cluster of rot,' what is referred to as 'the tumor.' However, according to Dr. Vivian Virginia Vetrano, who is a fasting expert (trained by the late Dr. Herbert M. Shelton, himself), "It often requires not one but two to three fasts" to achieve the desired results.

When the causes of cancer are discontinued, the body can redouble its efforts to detoxify itself of carcinogens and kill off aberrant cells which are parasites in the body.

Cancer, like the horse that is out of the corral, is a result of prior behaviors. The extent to which the situation can be redeemed depends upon the full set of circumstances. There is a point, naturally, when 'effects' are irreversible. We, often, cannot know when that point is upon us.

Recommended Readings (See also list of "References")

Results of one study conducted by the Medical School at the University of California, Los Angeles (UCLA) found that persons diagnosed "with cancer" who subscribe to conventional medical treatments survive approximately three years, as we have said; while those diagnosed and do not submit to conventional medical treatments survive an average of twelve and a half years. We also reported that 90% of the persons diagnosed with cancer do not, in fact, have cancer. You might want to avail yourself of the UCLA study.

Diet, Nutrition, and Cancer, a publication of the National Research Council of the National Academic of Sciences (1992), is especially recommended by Dr. T.C. Fry. He calls particular attention to Chapter 13, which reveals some of the many carcinogens that result from cooking foods.

My book, ***Helping Hand: A Guide to Healthy Living*** (as revised), is recommended as a basic wellness text, a fundamental guide to behaviors, eating habits and individual foods which are most conducive to living life in a manner which does not cause disease conditions to occur. Perhaps, most important about that book is how it lays out 'a transition program' for persons who make a decision and a commitment that they want, now, to take charge of their own health and well being.

Any book written by Dr. Herbert M. Shelton, "The Father of Natural Hygiene," is highly recommended. There are so many titles, one would be wise to start with a title which is closest to a present concern or personal interest.

John Tilden, M.D. has written, perhaps a classic small book that explains toxemia, the central element in the disease process, as also enumerated by Fry, Shelton, Burton, Diamond, Cinque, Allen, McDougall, and others.

Finally, as a companion to Dr. Shelton's ***Fasting Can Save Your Life,*** my book, ***Organic Wellness Fasting Technique,*** explores the term "therapeutic fasting" as a unique concept which requires guidance, both for effectiveness of the fast and for the safety and protection of the individual fasting. Erroneous fasting techniques can lead to serious outcomes. Individuals who want to supervise their own fasts should equip themselves with available and the most reliable information possible.

The body's own innate healing intelligence relies upon its own nerve energies to conduct its business, central of which is its own survival. A well-rested body handles most disease symptoms by routing waste elimination. During a sustained fast, the body is best able to corral its vital nerve energies to concentrate on its eliminative tasks, repair work and deferred maintenance.

Cancers, as other symptoms of "a crisis of toxemia," are the body's defensive steps to protect its tissues and organs from aberrant cells that have been impacted by carcinogens. *"Most cancer diagnoses," concludes Dr. T.C. Fry, "are only tumors or related sacs. The body can usually deal with these if afforded the opportunity—if causes are discontinued and healthful measures instituted."*

Toward a 'Cure' for Cancer

In the opinion of T.C. Fry, D. Sc., nothing would be more devastating to "the medical establishment than for someone to come up with a 'cure' for cancer." Surely, any such 'cure' would have an immediate financial impact on the income of physicians and the entire health care industry. However, that hypothetical blow to income flow would not likely be a deadly blow. After all, the medical profession and the health care establishment still have "conventional disease conditions and A.I.D.S.," which earn billions of dollars each year!

Furthermore, according to the New England Journal of Medicine (May 8, 1986), for more than thirty years, the medical profession has been "losing the war against cancer." Given all the research and treatment modalities available, "the most promising areas are in cancer prevention rather than treatment."

Prevention is best achieved through a vegetarian, raw foods, and healthful living lifestyle.

Prayer and a positive mental attitude notwithstanding, it is well to remember the survival rate for diagnosed persons who shun conventional medical treatment is 12.5 years, according to the UCLA study and but 3 years for those who submit to surgery, radiation, and/or chemotherapy.

Basic changes in the consumptive lifestyle of the diagnosed person are absolutely critical. Ancient wisdom constantly reminds us, if causes remain constant, so do effects. John Harris said at a wellness retreat in Cottonwood, Alabama: "If you keep on doing what you've been doing; you're going to keep on getting what you've been getting!"

Scientists did not find a cure for cancer because you don't go looking for rabbits at the tops of standing trees. Thirty years of spending billions of dollars and looking for the wrong things, in the wrong places, left researchers empty handed with no solution. Cancer, being an end pathology, remains illusive because doctors and researchers still fail to seek out the 'causes.'

Healthful Living the Best 'Treatment'

A thoughtfully directed and informed adaptation of a healthful living regimen could produce positive results in, perhaps, more than 90% of the diagnosed cases of cancer.

While an occasional latent effect will incapacitate the body, it is fair to say that what is referred to as 'pathology,' for example, has it origins in the 'third cause' of malfunction: from that which has been stored within the organism (or placed there directly). John H. Tilden, M.D. says, "The pathologic (organic change) panorama is one continuous evolution of intensifying effects" (***Toxemia***, 1926).

"Germs and other so-called causes may be discovered," he continued, "in the course of pathological development, but they are accidental, coincidental, or at most auxiliary—or, to use the vernacular of [law], obiter dicta." Dr. Tilden rejects the ancient notion that "evil spirits, germs, or so-called viruses cause the body to malfunction."

If, then, there is no external or 'outside cause' of body degeneration [disease]—excepting, of course, an act of God or the intervention of trauma—one can conclude that sickness or disease or body mal-function is a result of the evolutionary response [an 'effect'] to what the body has stored inside itself.

Put simply: one does not 'catch a cold or influenza,' but eventually 'comes down' with sickness due to poisonous substances lingering within the organism. Views of microorganisms from the vantage point of the microscope notwithstanding, a healthy body may be poisoned [traumatized], but as Dr. Tilden puts it, *"People do not get sick who have no bad habits!"* Of course, peoples of the world can and do become sick from external poisoning, unrelated to their personal behaviors.

Given the history of superstition, ignorance and demon worship, the past hundred years of "germ terror" have established a point of view that has been with us since childhood concerning disease and wellness, rooted in our historic fear of dying. It is not surprising, then, that when an entire association of "body caretakers" agrees that bodies "catch" different 'acute, chronic, and degenerative' diseases, the general public is 'programmed' to listen.

Only in recent times, when the same public has been demanding answers ***now*** to 'threats' to their lives by such monster afflictions as heart disease, cancer, and A.I.D.S. does there appear to be a flurry of equivocation, and the slow departure of individuals away from traditional "drug, cut and burn" treatment modalities.

Because of Universal Law, a body that has too long suffered the neglect of intolerable storage reaches a point ***['mid-life crisis']*** when the damage seems irreversible. ***Cause, whether recognized or not, guarantees effect.*** A body is created to return to its 'Creator' [is born to die]. Timing, to a great extent remains within the control of the organism [the individual]. In other words, a knowledge of the 'rule of Law' provides a rather clear focus on the preordained Order that follows the evolution of dynamic existence [life].

Put simply: if a body is able to use most of what is consumed, eliminate most of what it does not need, and store only what it desires for future use, "disease" is absent and such body lives out its fuller life with resolute wellness behaviors. Therefore, the proper response to the first sign of disease is to determine whether the cause is (1) act of Universal Law, (2) trauma, or (3) effect of internal storage. As we have suggested *perhaps as much as 95% of what we refer to as 'disease' emanates from body storage.*

Thus, it is immediately necessary to ascertain "how" Louise has been poisoning herself, or how she is being poisoned. There are seven possibilities, and these are channels of intake: food, drinks, air, chemicals, drugs, beliefs, and of course, Divine Providence (imperfections of Nature). These all are 'conduits' into the organism's reservoir, its 'storage tanks.'

Certainly, the simplistic basis of this discussion will come under attack from The Establishment. How else can it continue to justify billions of dollars in research expenditures? How else can the enviously high incomes of physicians [in particular] be maintained, if they are not "to save us—in our waning hours—from 'sudden, painful death' from chronic disease?"

You have no doubt heard someone say [or perhaps believe, yourself] that "They [the medical establishment] will have a cure in due course; so, I support the ...[A.I.D.S., Cancer, Arthritis, MS, Heart, etc.] Foundation." <u>Let the people know the whole truth</u>; and it shall set them free. Schopenhauer warns, however: "Convince a man against his will, he remains of the same opinion still."

The Time Clock of Life

Despite what we have been brought up believing, perhaps one concept is universally accepted, in some measure. That concept is that human life begins [at 6 'on the clock dial'], progresses through 12 'on the dial' [the height of maturity] and declines toward 6, again [where it "deep sixes," or dies]. This 'time clock of the life cycle' is inextricably tied to the Supreme Universal Law of "cause and effect." By maintaining our "normal body flora," we are told in ***The Merck Manual***, our organism remains healthy. However, by permitting 'enervation' [the build up of toxic stuff, caused by lifestyle interference of normal body elimination], disease symptoms appear, depending upon the organ, site, or intensity of 'the involvement.'

What all this means for the lay person is very simple: Whatever 'causes' disease symptoms is lethal or not, depending upon 'involvement' or intensity. In other words, not every one of Professor Peter Duesberg's 'recreational drugs' consumers will come down with 'A.I.D.S.' Nor will everyone who smokes cigarettes die from the debilitating habit. Alcoholics [cause] may even escape liver disease [effect]. However, since the Universal Law has been in place, no one escapes the impact of The Law. You and I may not "see" the unfolding drama [and what we "see" has been shown to not, necessarily, reflect 'reality'], but we can rest assured (for what that is worth) that the quality of life of the abused or enervated organism has been compromised, is being compromised, and shall be compromised.

Furthermore, whatever is believed, ultimately, concerning what is the 'cause' and what is the 'effect' of premature death, for sure, to avert it, ***corrective action must be instituted*** before the 'last tick' of the time clock. In Natural Hygiene, this process is known as 'internal cleansing,' an innate body function that I like referring to as 'organic ("therapeutic") fasting' [Also see Anderson, H. L. N., Organic Wellness Fasting Technique, BLI Publishers, Box 7219, Beverly Hills, CA 90212-7219, 1992, $9.95 (paper)].

Why Halt 'Premature' Death?

From a very selfish point of view, one wants to live longer when "life is the greater!" Some people view longevity as a condition of 'spirituality' that requires dedicated service to others. And, there are those who view life as "an unfair burden" which 'need not be extended, unnecessarily.' Still others, secretly and perhaps demonically motivated, might 'wish' premature death upon millions as a way to 'purge the human race' of lives considered 'burdensome' to the quality of life for the favored minority.

'People who care about wellness' [***Helping Hand: A Guide to Healthy Living***. United States, 1986; Nigeria, 1990; Germany, 1992; Japan 1994] have reasons for wanting to not only live longer, but to improve the quality of their lives and the lives of those to whom they reach out. These people are gripped in an endless struggle to 'free' themselves from perceptual limitations imposed by years of 'acculturation.' They have taken independent action to seek out and verify reliable information. Many of these individuals find their way to the 'doors of Natural Hygiene' literature.

When I was a student of religion at Yale University Divinity School in New Haven, Connecticut, Professor H. Richard Niehbur told us that, as seminarians and theologians, our task was not to solve all the problems of humankind, rather it was "to raise the right questions." Much of my life, since 1957-1959, has been spent attempting to free my mind processes such that I could 'receive perceptions' which differ in kind and substance from 'the stuff' we are, ordinarily, fed in the public media and in educational institutions. By so doing, I come closer to raising "the right questions." In this writing, I share that YDS legacy with you.

Challenge to "See" The 'Causes'

This book is a challenge "to see the causes" of our disease conditions. By learning to look for causes, and not being distracted by 'descriptions of the effects,' or by symptoms and developing symptoms of ultimate effects, we place ourselves in a position ***to remain empowered*** or to restore our empowerment. When we can, clearly, trace back to the source of our poisoning, we can further 'quantify' our toxic storage. What, for example would be the source of the poisoning [the cause] if by the year 2020 "some people" 'wished for' the demise of half the world's population [the effect]? Now, we are focusing on 'cause.' Who for example had most to gain from the orchestrated death of Princess Diane? Who from inter-regional or other "violent attacks?" Half the world's population 'must die' by the year 2020?

In this manner, we can look, specifically, at 'counter measures' which have application for our, individual, "toxemia" [assuming there is personal confirmation of Natural Hygiene's central thesis: ***'all diseases are the same disease.'***] Most people who suffer disease will need to learn a proper and safe method of fasting.' A thorough knowledge of fasting, from the research and clinical evidence of Natural Hygiene, provides a reasonable indication of a 'recommended' course of action (Shelton, ***Fasting Can Save Your Life***, http://organicwellness.com or http://www.amazon.com).

Not only that, other realistic possibilities emerge. One is able to ascertain for oneself: (1) what 'kind' of fasting to do; (2) how long to fast; (3) how frequently to fast; and (4) what are the most favorable environmental circumstances in which to carry on one's fasting. Equally important, one comes to better understand how important it is to immediately cease all forms of poisonous intake or consumption—especially of drugs or medications—in conjunction with a fundamental change in philosophy and in lifestyle.

Overall, 'a wellness profile' is constructed in the mind, and eventually is implemented into the individual's lifestyle. For, it becomes ever so clear that those already impacted by actual, or believed, disease conditions will need to assist the organism in its elimination work. That is one positive step; another is to provide the additional support the body needs: organically grown, raw foods, pure water, sunshine, exercise, clean air, positive belief structures, reliable information and loving environmental factors.

Peoples with melanin, in all parts of the world, have real concerns for the ailments they witness around them—and rightly so! They will need to follow a chosen path. Of course, we in Natural Hygiene suggest this kind of process: (1) arm yourself with reliable information [information which, among other things, meets the 'common sense' test]; (2) accept the fact that there is no 'quick fix,' but that the restoration of health must be as deliberate as the destruction of health ["things equal to the same thing are equal to each other," in this case, individual actions and their results]; (3) recognize that some afflicting toxemia is a result of actions not your own [such as military, work place, pharmaceutical and chemical poisoning]; (4) design a wellness lifestyle (which works for you and is consistent with the literature); (5) implement regular—and sometimes long term—fasting into your wellness lifestyle regimen; (6) observe proven 'rules of wellness,' which are, in fact, the basic tenets of a healthful lifestyle; (7) and finally, always question or disbelieve what you are 'told,' because we have proven over and over again that "things are not what they seem!"

There is plenty of company around, others who have similar anxieties, concerns and objectives; and, there are many that can offer support, assistance and reassurances that individually designed wellness routines are, in fact, consistent with current research and practice within Natural Hygiene. To access these unlimited resources, one might write to the American Natural Hygiene Society of Canada, or to Organic Wellness Crusade, PO Box 7219, Beverly Hills, California, 90212-7219. Visit the Web Site at http://www.organicwellness.com or email to: truth@organicwellness.com. Or, one might want to look up the Healthful Living Institute at www.healthfullivingintl.com.

Individual donations to either organization help further the dissemination of Hygienic and reliable information.

Chapter Six

A.I.D.S. from a Natural Hygiene Perspective

Understanding the nature of "Acquired Immune Deficiency Syndrome" hinges upon public acceptance of four contributing factors: (1) the build up of chemicals and pesticides from the food chain in the human organism; (2) early consumption of over-the-counter, prescription, and illegal drugs; (3) accumulated carcinogens from cooked, deranged and 'fast foods;' and (4) synergistic effects (the effects of chemicals interacting with each other within the human organism). This latter phenomenon is, perhaps, the single most deadly [and 'required'] variable in A.I.D.S., as opposed to cancer *(which has its genesis in the food chain)*, for example.

Synergistic effects are little known partly because there are too many contingent variables. We will speak more about these later. For now, let's consider what might be called "the McDonald-Domino Syndrome" (my reference to the pattern of luring very young children into the fast food dragnet, and all other age groups up to the most senior among us!).

The build up, in the intestinal tract, of the effects from accumulated food supply pesticides; putrefaction and carcinogens from cooked foods; work place, military, and environmental pollutants; consumption of antibiotics, medications, alcohol, and so called 'recreational drugs;' and the dynamic or synergistic effects of these various combinations impact the body's entire immune network such that lethal conditions result. Neither scientific research nor medical practice is either sufficiently aware of, or remotely knowledgeable to diagnose, let alone pretend to treat these effects. This is why hysteria, pain, suffering, despair, or death often results for those accepting the 'AIDS' diagnosis and mind-set.

Perhaps it becomes clearer why such a medical scramble to identify, pinpoint, and epitomize "AIDS" took place in the early 1980's, first blaming the homosexual community, then the vast continent of Africa, then sexual and 'body fluids' exchanges. This "rush to judgment" is to be expected by those who control what the public knows and is encouraged to believe. This explains why 'human icons'—actors, athletes, famous people—are generally used as 'spokespersons' to tell the public what to believe. And the public buys into it!

Professor Peter Duesberg, microbiologist at the University of California Berkeley, postulates that, "There are two new phenomena present among us since 1980: the use of 'recreational drugs' and the incidence of AIDS; and both of these occur within the same populations." Duesberg, perhaps more than any other, draws our collective attention to the 'outward and visible signs' of the internal and biological dynamics present as the synergistic effects incapacitate the body's immune system (gradually kill off white blood cells until too few are left for effective 'defense' of the organism). This is why, perhaps, "smoking pot" is such a 'pleasant' death trap: it takes so much longer to happen, by then "nobody really gives a damn!" Of course, the notion that health consequences from pot smoking "are deferred" is a pure deception. What happens, as with Santa Claus and the chimney, pot smokers 'believe' their health problems are related to other factors. A favorite one of which is "heredity." ***Only the son or the daughter of a pot smoker can make such claim, and only in the first generation!***

Why AIDS Is So Deadly

The deadly consequences of A.I.D.S. simply explain medical confusion, public panic, hysterical demands for "a cure," and the opportunistic appearance on the market of various drugs such as AZT (none of which can reverse the synergistic effects of damage already done).

What drugs, in what amounts, interact with what other drugs and toxins, in what amounts, under what types of host conditions, under what circumstances, over what periods of time, and of what intensity? Obviously, there are these and other variables which when medical science eventually admits to existing, would still confound conventional medical wisdom, giving rise to even greater abuse of drugs and pharmaceuticals, and of the conventional medical therapies of surgery, radiation, and chemotherapy. ***Abstaining from drugs is the public's best hope!***

When treatments 'work,' it suggests two possibilities: One, the person was incorrectly diagnosed, as many are; and/or, Two, other non-medical changes in the individuals' lifestyles were sufficiently consistent with the principles of Natural Hygiene to allow the body to effectively accomplish its eliminative and reparative tasks, thus healing itself (as only the body can do).

The typical misdiagnosis—which sets up the metal devastation—occurs when an individual 'testing positive' for the so-called "HIV virus" is permitted to believe that this body defensive posture is actually the forerunner to the onset of the 'dreaded disease.' The implication is that there is a scientific or actual relationship between the 'test results' and the ultimate collapse of the immune system that could lead to eventual death.

HIV, A Body Defensive Effort?

In fact, what is called the "HIV virus" is an antibody response to new threats within the body created by the various chemical substances interacting with or against each other, disrupting normal body function, and potentially incapacitating essential organs, despite the body's attempts to survive this onslaught.

This antibody presence, itself, never leads to the absolute "crisis of toxemia" we have come to know as AIDS. This phenomenon is not inconsistent with how John H. Tilden, M.D. might describe "Acquired Immune Deficiency Syndrome."

In short, too many people are dying prematurely; and too few of us ever discover why they are dying! Until we can identify the 'causes' of death, we are hopelessly unable to have real impact upon the 'effects' [too much suffering, reduced quality of living, and unnecessary death]. The fact of the matter is, however, that we do have a choice! All we have to do is exercise our options and select the alternatives favorable to us and to our wellness.

"What If…?" Scenario on 'HIV/AIDS in Africa'

When an aroused public—or an individual—fails to comprehend or to receive 'comfortable' explanations, speculation often sets in. I have said before, we who write are very much like you, those who read what is written. While on her trip to Los Angeles in the first two months of 2001, I handed to former First Lady of South Africa, Dr. Winnie Mandela, the following "What If…?" writing:

'Tell me not in mournful numbers,
'Life is but an empty dream….'
For the soul is dead that slumbers…
And, things are not what they seem.
—From Henry Wadsworth Longfellow's Psalm of Life

'If what is revealed to me is true—and I believe it is—and caring people in the world do not act responsibly, may God have mercy on our lost souls! If "thinking peoples" cannot see through the thickness of the "HIV/AIDS hype," who can expect victims to ever know what assailed them? Or, for non-victims to know the truth?

'WHAT IF…the U.S. campaign to save the declining funding for cancer research, which after more than 30 years only saw

increases in cancer deaths, catapulted into history's largest ever "funding for research jackpot," the "HIV/AIDS' construct?

'WHAT IF...Dr. T. C. Fry, Prof. Peter Duesberg, (myself), and many others are correct: "HIV does not, and indeed cannot 'cause' anything;" and AIDS is the 'flip side of poisoning from drugs and chemicals, and from nothing else (dying from poisoning, malnutrition, starvation, and drugs looks the same)?

'WHAT IF...the motivation behind lying to the world were: 1) Money, some $15 billion a year, and growing; 2) Population control, the wanton killing of millions in strategic locations, camouflaging racism and economic greed; 3) World domination, of individuals and of nations—killing and terrorizing masses of peoples, destabilizing their homelands, turning humans into refugees (who can no longer farm to feed themselves!); and nations, by pressing them into a bottomless pit dependency on buying drugs (emptying their national treasuries!) to "cure" what only clean water, nutritious food, and an anti-chemical warfare strategy can prevent?

WHAT IF...billions of dollars donated "for HIV/AIDS research" (even) by well-meaning donors were really fueling the clandestine campaigns to dislodge families and disrupt national economics, especially on the African continent?

'WHAT IF...Africa "falls" to the control of "foreign interests," which "dark continent" will be next? Will it be India? Will it be China? Will it be South America? Will it be the Pacific Rim? If "this thing" succeeds, who will be next?

'WHAT IF...the money now spent in HIV/AIDS research and HIV/AIDS treatments were spent on purifying drinking water; providing nutritious foods; demilitarizing regions; reining in chemical warfare; and encouraging organic farming; and making comfortable those who might be too poisoned already to completely recover?

'WHAT IF...you and I wake up (tomorrow) and there are no refugees, no malnutrition, no starvation, no "recreational" or otherwise "forced" drug usage, no air-borne killer chemicals descending, no military campaigns being fueled, do you think

you or I could find a single incident of HIV/AIDS? Wherein would there be profit? Is HIV/AIDS any less a deliberate creation than are forms of credit?

'WHAT IF...FUNDING FOR HIV/AIDS STOPPED TOMORROW, ALSO? WHO WOULD SUFFER THE GREATEST FINANCIAL LOSS? YOU WANT MOTIVE, MEANS, METHODS, ACCESS, AND ALIBI? YOU'VE GOT ALL!'

Letter to Black Preachers [Faith-Based Initiative]

March 7, 2002

Bishop Harold Calvin Ray
Founder/CEO, Redemptive Life Fellowship
West Palm Beach, Florida

Re: A Divine Warning?

Dear Bishop Ray:

Recently, I received a colorful brochure featuring eleven "black preachers" and in the twelfth spot, posters of National Civil Rights Museum and Denny's. I wondered, "Are these twelve reminiscent of the "Original Twelve?" Going farther, as the brochure invited, I visited www.civilrightsmuseum.org. Behind the obvious, my attention was drawn to the not-too-obvious:

1. You eleven "black preachers" sit as the Board of Governors of the **National Center for Faith Based Initiative**. That sounds like the pro-president Bush church funding campaign. When government funds, government 'controls,' or seriously influences (building up a terminal dependency upon!).
2. Looking at the eleven members of The Board of Governors, conservatively speaking, you Governors

influence - in a significant manner - perhaps some 20 million people of color in this country, alone. Your influence over other races, and over non-Americans cannot be measured. That's valuable influence!

3. Twenty million represents, perhaps, 35% to 45% of all people classified as African Americans (see www.WashitawNation.com) in the United States of America.
4. Denny's - while conceivably "better than McDonald's, Burger King, Chuck E. Cheeze, or Domino's Pizza - has to viewed, nonetheless in the category of a "fast food restaurant," at least to the extent Denny's generally serves up the S.A.D. (Standard American Diet), reportedly **the major cause of cancer** in Western Society, and the number one killer of children in America!

Back to President Bush's "faith-based initiative." Many knowledgeable people believe there is a connection between this administration's funding of "black churches" and the "slow down in new cases of A.I.D.S. among black Americans." Some believe Mr. Bush's motive is to "increase testing for A.I.D.S. among African Americans!"

It appears that "there is a deadly virus going around; and African Americans are more susceptible, or so THEY would have us believe. You might even conclude, with many others that A.I.D.S. testing is a good thing!" What is not obvious, however, is that the more people get tested for A.I.D.S., the more " new cases of A.I.D.S." are reported in the press. "Sure," you might even conclude, "testing is how people discover whether or not they have 'caught' the A.I.D.S./HIV [virus]!"

Let us look, again, at the "virus theory." That a deadly virus is going around would be the obvious conclusion [albeit well programmed]. ***The not-so-obvious fact is that what most of the "new cases " have in common is that they were all tested sometime earlier*** (or, otherwise, are linked to drugs/medicines). Now, let's say I made up a poison to "kill niggers," and I got medical people to label my poison, "H.I.V./A.I.D.S." What better way for me to get my poison into the bodies of my intended victims! Yes, I think you are beginning to get my drift, Of course, I would not poison everyone being tested - just an increasingly significant number, slowly upping the percentage as my test population increases (thanks to my friends over at the National Center for Faith Based Initiative)!

Bishop, can you recall your activities during the past four years? Are you aware that during that same period of time, some 4 million blacks have quietly died ["of A.I.D. S."] in South Africa, alone, approximately 20% of the black population? In 100,000 years of history, these black people –our Muurish cousins– lived on their lands, dying natural deaths. In the recent era, somebody else wants their lands, and their natural resources! So, these ancient land-owners become the "victims of new, killer viruses [poisons]!"

A new "low income labor force" is replacing African Americans; so, they, too, are becoming "expendable." Drugs (illicit, prescription, over-the-counter), street violence, poor health, denatured foods, traditional diseases, auto deaths, gang murders, police murders - all of these fail to compensate for the fact that **the white race's reproduction rate is now an increasingly negative statistic**! With a Radio Shack calculator, a grade school child can figure out at what year, in the future, there will be no more white people!

Have you figured it out yet? **A.I.D.S. is a military weapon!** We are in a "war" for our very survival! Churches are critical to the strategy of "the enemy" (see,"Interview with T. C. Fry" at www@organicwellness.com). How else can these millions of "sheep" be led "to the slaughter," without arousing suspicion? How many inches of newsprint have you read in the past four years about just the 4 million South African deaths? Do you have any idea of the total number of "black deaths" during the same period of time?

"Kill 'em and/or bankrupt their national treasuries!" That is the "win-win strategy." It is about **control**. The "honey" of control is human greed--the ultimate capital "sin" in the history of the low-melanin community (*The Nature and Purpose of Disease: Definitive Guide for Peoples with Melanin*, $23.95+SH/319pp, American University Publishers, P.O. Box 4277, Inglewood, Calif. 90309-4277; see also www. WashitawNation.com).

In the ancient game of dominoes invented by our ancestors, there is a saying: "Not all money is good money!" Your Board of Governors is playing a high-stakes game. Who is going to win? The record shows Jesus was a black man, and his mother, too, was black--even his father. Moses was black and so were the Israeli. What would wide spread knowledge of **this truth** do to the image of the Christian Church, I wonder?

Shepherds of your Christian flocks, this message to you is simple: (1) **keep your people out of "A.I.D.S. testing programs**," as a first step; (2) **support African leaders who are aware of The Great A.I.D.S Hoax** (T.C. Fry, 1987); and, (3) learn and teach the truth [that promises to "set you free!"] as a continuing objective.

Faithfully Her Servant,

Henry L.N. Anderson, B.S., M.A.R., Ed.D.,D.D.
Author, *The Nature and Purpose of Disease*

Cc: Bishop Charles E. Blake
Bishop J. Delano Ellis, II

Bishop Floyd Flake
Bishop T.D. Jakes
Bishop Eddie Long
Bishop Andrew Merritt
Bishop Paul S. Morton
Bishop Gilbert E. Patterson
Bishop Carlton E. Pearson
Bishop Mack Timberlake
Her Imperial Highness, Verdiacee "Tiari" Washitaw-Turner Goston El-Bey

[Edited slightly for inclusion in this book.]

Diseases and Disorders

In his own chapter, Dr. Fry presents his argument—with which this writer concurs—establishing why humans are anatomically ***frugivorous*** and how following "our natural disposition" humans can live a life that is sickness and disease free.

"Dis-ease" in the human organism is symptomatic, i.e., it is evidence of the body's own efforts to survive beyond conditions it finds intolerable. These symptoms are called by various names depending upon their severity, prevailing characteristics and location. Examples are lung disease, kidney disease, heart disease, stomach disease, "female troubles," and so forth.

Disorders, on the other hand, reflect distress conditions brought on by other direct and/or indirect causes. For example, diabetes is a condition usually brought on by the body's inability to produce sufficient insulin. Overweight, over consumption of starches and carbohydrates, overeating, lack of exercise, stress, consumption of alcohol and/or of other sugars are associated causes of diabetes. In reality, the terms are practically interchangeable.

Genetic Diseases: An Illusion?

Children, born to parents exposed to alcohol, drugs, military and workplace toxins, tobacco products, sugars, 'fast foods' and a variety of coffee-tea-soft drink and other beverages, are often born with various disorders such as, muscular dystrophy, leukemia, "HIV and full-blown AIDS," organ "diseases," ear-eye-throat and nose disorders, certain types of deformities [also often related to over-the-counter and prescription medications taken by one and/or both parents], and even diabetes with the infant body's inability to produce insulin. *Western society 'blames' the mother; in most such cases, **however, it is most likely the father who is the culprit!***

So-called "genetic diseases" are <u>one-generation disorders</u> brought on by the consumptive conditions of the host or parental bodies. *Such conditions, whether midget structure or limb deformity, are limited to one generation.* Healthful consumption by the deformed child will guarantee a healthy offspring, assuming both parents were healthy. In other words, a midget marrying a normal person will produce a normal child, assuming neither parent indulged abusive behaviors themselves.

This brief discussion is not intended to be exhaustive nor exclusionary, but only to illustrate the difference between 'classical diseases' and disorders, as these might stem from quite varied and different causes. A reference to a condition as "a disease" does not make it so. Disease describes an enervated state brought on by un-eliminated wastes or toxemia; disorders describe 'accidents,' deprivation and trauma. Therefore, remedial approaches are likewise different. These matters are discussed in more detail in following chapters.

Chapter Seven

HIV/AIDS: Is There a Political Dimension?

What if...by taking the so-called "AIDS test," an individual comes under the 'magic' of the AIDS phenomenon? That is to say, what if in the process of, and under guise of being tested, individuals *really* are being administered "the poison?" After all, it is quite well known that the more AIDS testing that goes on, the more "cases of HIV/AIDS" are reported! Coincidental, or the 'expected' results from 'better health care?' You decide. Meanwhile, let's follow the "argument."

Not everyone gets the lethal potion! It is not necessary to poison all—just enough to keep "the disease" flourishing. The more people are 'tested,' the more people will—at a time in the future—"come down with" what will be, effectively, "full blown AIDS."

The "magic" works; the 'slight of hand' occurs. The public is <u>not</u> the wiser; the stage is set; the results are predictable; the people are sacrificed (martyred) for two reasons: 1) their demise is a 'population-control' device; and 2) in their becoming sick and dying, a "great financial whirlwind" is guaranteed for the pharmaceutical cartel that produces the "expensive drugs *needed* to treat—and possibly 'cure' or stop—this "dreaded pandemic" that is "spreading like a wild fire, out of control!"

While 'testing' for and treating of so-called HIV/AIDS are the principle "causes" of the effects, compelling large numbers of people to take the so-called "AIDS test" (unlawfully?)

guarantees the 'random selection' of a "sufficient number of future HIV/AIDS cases!" No one should be forced to submit to AIDS testing!

Any such criminal assault on the world's population—a political dimension—must be stopped; or, *the genocide and human carnage* will go unabated into the dismal future. The 21st Century will come to be known as the "Age (Century) of the 'Human Purge!'"

HIV/AIDS As a 'Military Weapon'

In a press conference hosted by my friends, Dr. Clark and Dr. Jeannette Parker, at the Beverly Hills Hotel, this writer asked the President of the Central African Republic (*Republique Centrafricaine*), Son Excellence Ange Felix Patasse, whether he had considered "HIV/AIDS in Africa" to be suspect, given the book on the subject by T. C. Fry and the public positions taken by Prof. Peter Duesberg of the University of California at Berkeley, and others. President Patasse responded: "I am not a doctor; so, I will defer such matters to those who are doctors. But, whatever 'causes' AIDS, we must stop its spread!" To that I could not agree more!

Few African countries, but a good number of other countries, as reported in the press, have engaged in the use of so-called "chemical weapons." Take note that "The Gulf War Syndrome" (10 years after chemical warfare was used) is now known and accepted. In the future, the world can anticipate the "outbreak of AIDS in Iraq," as "the pandemic" finds its way to the home base of 'public enemy number one, Saddam Hussein' (as former President George Bush would have the world believe). This is especially probable now that "Junior Bush" is back in the White House, with Gen. Colin Powell as his Secretary of State!

An international "military complex" is most comfortable with AIDS as an 'international pandemic.' Public sensitivity has been deadened; ***and millions are being "put to death"*** (from a distance, and under the cover of "disease epidemic," the same disinformation strategy as 'Hitler's Big Lie!'). There is no direct assault, no bombs being dropped, and no military personnel put at apparent risk. It's all very neat.

The 'Big Lie' principle still works. It works because the lie is believed. Belief quickly turns a genius into a fool. And, even people of good will (as were many Germans in Nazi Germany, and Allies in other nations!) are prone to act, based on personal motivation, from the desire to be rich to the most fundamental desire to remain alive! Nor can any of us be absolutely certain; however, we err when we do not act on our "gut perceptions." Certainly, I am not looking for 'validation.' I believe.

The world's population co-conspires by default with the military cartel by believing, first and foremost, in the propaganda that there exists in our world "an enemy." Without *an enemy* there is little justification for a military to exist—weak or strong! And, this armed minority perceives 80% of the world's population (*peoples with melanin*) as the real enemy!

"The AIDS pandemic" becomes a military tactic "to neutralize and control" the enemy (those with dominant genes containing melanin). As with clandestine schemes throughout history, "the AIDS epidemic" strategy must also fail—even as a military strategy. It will fail as did, and will, its forebears because the perpetrators fail to grasp the simple truth: *there is only oneness in human Creation.*

Consider this: peoples with the darkest melanin—black people—can produce all other hues of people; but, no other hue can produce black people! What military strategists—even quantum physicists and religious advocates—very well understand is that humans differ from animals, not so much in the level of their intelligence, but in the fact that <u>only humans have the ability to exercise 'belief' over 'reason</u>.'

Advertisers know this fundamental characteristic of the human condition. It is by employing this principle the late Senator Joseph McCarthy could convince Americans that they were in imminent danger from "Communists within our national government." Or, it helps explain why Americans are led to believe that "AIDS comes from Africa!" Or, why a well-organized advertising campaign can sell millions of dollars worth of "pet rocks," and get anti-drug advocates to "advertise" the very product they are against, by having them paste on their auto bumpers, advertisement stickers that read: "Just say NO to drugs!" "Madison Avenue knows to whom they pitch," said US Presidential candidate, Dr. John Hagelin in his May 11, 2000 lecture in Chapel Hill, North Carolina.

What Personal Danger Is There for Me?

When 'threats' are imminent, everyone wants to know: "Am I in danger?" If you are an individual with melanin, part of 80% of the world's population, the answer is, "Yes," you are in danger! If, on the other hand, you are an individual in the minority, among 20% of the world's population (*which is no longer reproducing itself*), you, too, are in danger!

In the former instance the threat is from without; it is orchestrated by sinister minds that believe in their "prior" claim to the resources of the earth: space, water, air, mineral, vegetable, and animal (including human). In the latter instance, the threat is from within. It is the result of estrangement, of persisting in maintaining the presence of an "enemy," thus separating the Natural Oneness of Creation. People without melanin ("white people")—no matter how ingenious or how dull-witted—tend to believe they are superior creatures. They believe their perceived intelligence makes them so. They "prove" their thesis by omission and by selectively comparing institutions they create with institutions created by their (acknowledged) majority—*peoples with melanin.*

Let us look more into this 'illusionism.' A national 'system' of school buses carry children back and forth, maintaining the "illusion of an enemy," but in fact, continues to nurture and imbed a larger system of the separation of the races, of the classes, of the oneness of peoples (America being a "melting pot").

If Americans 'refuse' (by some unseen, unknown, improbable eventuality) to accept "homelessness" as a 'necessary evil' in modern society, they could no longer accept AIDS overseas, or cancer at home as "necessary evils" as well.

What happens to people—politically—stems from what they endorse militarily, and that 'attitude' translates into what is conceivable in matters of public health and personal wellness. All constructs depend upon the notion that some people are more 'blessed,' or more 'cursed' than others; that a thing called 'disease' visits the least worthy, except in other instances where people contract the "expected disease condition."

We have been taught to "expect" AIDS, for example; to expect "terrorism from extremists;" to expect "human rights violations" overseas, but not IRS or FBI or law enforcement violations of human rights here at home. Why, as another example, should anyone ever consider that courts across America have always seen "justice" differently for persons with melanin?

If these "slight of hand" realities were not so similarly construed, perhaps it could be argued that "a child catches a cold," or that the military campaigns across Africa and other parts of the world are as naturally a consequence of peoples' inability to co-exist as AIDS is the "natural" consequence of "HIV."

But, we cannot succumb to such deceptive constructs because we know too well the consequences of driving a motor vehicle without regard for traffic signals! We know too that jumping from atop a building is likely to result in serious injury or death. There is no particular industrial (monetary) interest in those examples of *cause and effect.* When it comes to meat, dairy, alcoholic beverages, tobacco products, religion, health care (responding to sickness, primarily), and even the production and marketing of other foods and beverages, vested interests promote their own self interests, not the public welfare! Politicians—whether public or military—tend to do the same!

Enter "Madison Avenue," the genius of marketing, the "image makers." Their job is made easier because we 'learned' early in life that "the stork delivered the baby!" We are well taught in believing what is *not* true. The "germ theory" and a belief in "contagion" form the 'handcuffs' that restrain, and a manipulated public continues—long after the 'cuffs' are removed—to believe and respond to "pre-conditioning" (just as the elephant that will not move farther than the length of *its former* restraining chain)!

So it is that, "For lack of knowledge my children perish." I stopped by a farmers' market in search of something tempting. Imagine that "I saw an animal that sounded like a goat, gave milk like a cow, but fluttered huge wings like a chicken!" So much for "genetically engineered" foods! And, so much for the much advertised and publicized notion of, "HIV, the virus that causes AIDS!" Both of the foregoing statements are "equally true." Believe what you will.

But, if you are simply curious, or fancy yourself a history buff, watch out for the following developments: Under the 2001 Bush Administration, an imminent world class "threat to national security" will be identified, publicized and demonized. This "enemy" will give impetus to massive military build-up (the spending of hundreds of billions for a "strong and prepared national defense!"). Congress will vote in favor of spending the dollars because the public will concur (having been convinced the 'threat is imminent to their own personal safety!').

Hundreds—perhaps even thousands—will die ("honorably," of course—from whatever national perspective!) And, as regretful as it is, and as painful, to have to witness these unfortunate deaths of women, old people, children, unborn infants and military personnel, these deaths will dwarf those that shall occur in the name of the so-called "AIDS pandemic!" There will be reports of "new and deadlier strains of the virus."

The one tragedy in all of the above will be the level at which people believe. In anticipating the massive dying in the name of the "virus-disease paradigm," I must conclude: God must be wrought with us humans, and will probably "punish" us by making the world all one race. Then, I quickly recall that

Iranians and Iraqis are one race, yet they kill each other; North Koreans and South Koreans are one race, yet they killed each other; Irish Protestants and Irish Catholics are one race, yet they kill each other. Palestinians and Israelis are one race; they kill each other, and there is no lasting peace!

So, I become keenly aware: one race-ness is not the answer. But to face the challenge of decency—that is the issue. God will continue to offer humankind challenges. Some of us will meet these "challenges" so boldly as to sit upon them and have our lunch. Others will be sat upon by the very "challenges," and they shall be the lunch! So, we do have a choice; and this "right to choose" is consistent with Natural Law, the law of "effects of cause."

Nonetheless, some of you—as do I—pain for the families, and for the friends, who experience the personal now-sadness of witnessing the demise of one individual (or of millions!), attributed to AIDS, no matter what the 'politics' of AIDS are. Your pay, too, is real; and the loss you experience is immediate. You, too, might become burdened by your sense of helplessness. Perhaps, the ultimate AIDS tragedy is when peoples of the world believe what they are told, and raise too little objection to the pillage. The world's peoples must respond, as Son Excellence Ange Felix Patasse, Presidente de Republique Centrafricaine, urges a civilized society: "...Whatever 'causes' AIDS, we must stop its spread!" The solution must match the problem; it must be political as opposed to 'medical.' A "motive" for AIDS is the money derived from drugs/chemicals; the remedy must be organized action of the peoples of the world. We best know such action as that conducted by representative governments, "in the peoples' best interests." Herein lies Africa's unique role in saving much of the human race from 'orchestrated' annihilation, as a model for the rest of the peoples with melanin to follow.

Passion, religious beliefs, humanitarian concern notwithstanding, the "commercial aspect" of AIDS might have slipped our attention. *In the global marketplace, the combined value of diamonds, crude oil, and gold may not equal the potential revenue generation of AIDS pharmaceuticals, if world governments succumb to the propaganda and blackmail machines behind the so-called "AIDS pandemic!"*

In refusing to endorse the use of AZT for pregnant women in South Africa (population control—and more!), despite international pressures President Mbeki said publicly, "The (AIDS) debate seems to be fueled by the discussion of buying more and more drugs—not what to do to address these basic problems" (*L.A. Watts Times*, June 1, 2000). In response, "five major drug companies have offered to cut the price of HIV and AIDS treatments." But even at reduced prices, President Mbeki observed, the cost of such drugs would be so prohibitive that "it would consume the totality of the government's health budget," President Mbeki protested.

Unless world governments see the picture clearly, countries will be, literally, "owned by" the pharmaceutical cartel, much like individuals are turned into 'persons' or "personal property of the states in which they are domiciled, when their certificates of birth are filed." AIDS is part and parcel of a larger "disease." That disease is called ***human greed***!

Chapter Eight

Addiction: Most Subtle of "Diseases?"

Addiction can be described as 'persistent affinity for substance/s that provide no nutritive value to the body.' *Addiction*, itself, claims far more lives and good health than do the more recognized addictions of alcohol and drugs. And, these 'other addictions' are by far more commonplace, even if less recognized. People become addicted to sugar, salt, tobacco, pepper, caffeine, bicarbonate of soda (as in soft drinks), nicotine, desserts, bread, cereals, medications, cooked foods, oily chips, and the general fare we all recognize as "fast foods."

Flesh eating is both physically and psychologically 'addictive.' Non-flesh-eating humans tend to be well; experience fewer disease conditions; and live longer, higher quality lives than their counterparts. Nor do we need to over illustrate the point: substances that "taste good" generally are altered substances and are, most often, not very high on the list of quality foods for peoples who want to maintain wellness, including a higher quality of life.

Psychological factors that interfere with normal body functioning—persistently engaged—are psychic addictions whose effects are, perhaps, even more lethal than conventional 'addictive substances.' What Dr. Shelton and others cite over and over again as 'moods' or 'emotions' (even belief structures) disrupt and negate normal body functions, negatively affecting organs and overall well being of the organism.

In short, mental addiction is, possibly, more detrimental than is "substance addiction." Many cancer deaths occur in people who harbored a passionate hatred for sometime before—and leading into—their demise.

When it comes to 'conventional addiction,' almost everyone knows someone whose family has been impacted by the high cost of addiction. Lives have been "put on hold," as my nephew, Kevin, complained upon residing with his alcohol-abused father after the death of his mother and family financial security had been compromised; children's futures have been sacrificed; and potentially productive individuals have had their potential reduced to 'surviving the next high.' Given this dismal scenario, what the public needs access to is a program or method of over coming the addiction—no matter to what! Thus, following the principles of Natural Hygiene, a workable program is suggested below.

Addiction Reversal Program

What follows is an "eight-day" program for reversing debilitating addictions. It is also true that fasting for thirty days, on water only, will 'free' one from most addictive urges. However, not many people are well-trained enough to manage such a long period of fasting. Nor is it recommended, really! I have knowledge of individuals who have taken themselves through a rehabilitative abstinence period to such an extent they were able to overcome their former 'dependency.' Below is an alternative program that 'ordinary' peoples might employ in dealing with their addictions.

Day One

Drink down one pint of fresh bottled grape juice during an hour or so, first thing after water in the morning. Expect to make one or more 'bathroom calls!' Once the stomach seems settled (approximately 1-2 hours later), drink down one pint of fresh vegetable juice over a period of one hour.

Sip one full glass of H.A.R.A./tm (Hurdle Antechachexy Regenerative Agent, an organic cactus prickly pear juice extract in 99% distilled water) as you would cool water. One or two hours later, "chew" down another 8-to-12 oz of H.A.R.A. Before retiring, drink by 'chewing' another glass of cranberry or cranberry cocktail juice. At bedtime, drink one 8-oz glass of H.A.R.A./tm.

Note: H.A.R.A. is an organically grown and produced wellness body tonic that allows the body to cleanse itself with minimum interference. It is marketed exclusively by its manufacturer, http://www.organicwellness.com.

Day Two

Within half hour of awakening, drink one 8-oz class of H.A.R.A. Within another half hour, if there is no bowel movement drink 8-oz of grape juice. In fifteen minutes, drink another 8-oz, but do so slowly, chewing each "swallow" as you drink.

Continue until there is at least one bowel movement, or a quart of grape juice has been consumed. Resume drinking H.A.R.A. as you would regular water (only do so in a "chewing" fashion).

By early afternoon of Day 2, any sensation of 'hunger" or the desire to eat should have faded. For twenty (20) minutes, meditate in a warm, quite place, focusing on the body's "desperate cleansing activity" to get rid of poisons and any excess of acids.

Drink H.A.R.A. until bedtime. Just before retiring, tell yourself—aloud—"I am becoming clean. It is working. What I am doing is working to get me clean." Go to bed smiling.

Day Three

Upon arising, drink 8-oz of distilled water. In 30 minutes have your first glass of H.A.R.A.

Meditate for 20 minutes. Repeat to yourself, "I am becoming clean." Say this over and over and over in your mind. Smile. Feel yourself smiling.

When you go to the toilet to relieve your bowels, try never to 'push down,' but rather 'suck-up or pull in your stomach muscles. Allow your bowels to empty as freely and easily as is natural for your system. Do not become anxious. It is quite "normal" to have three or four "easy bowel movements" per day. Also, you might not have any!

Plan out in your head what physical activities you will do, for from 30 to 45 minutes. Move into these activities slowly, with joy and anticipation. As you engage this "work-out" repeat these words: "I am becoming clean. It is working. What I am doing is working to get me clean."

Freely express gratitude to the "God" of your religion, or of your 'memory.' Give thanks and praises. Acknowledge the assistance and support of others. Thank "God" for the kindness of friends and family, and for the thoughtfulness of 'strangers.'

Rest in the late morning, early afternoon, and early evening. These rest periods can be short or long, so long as they do not cause you to remain up too late in the evening. It is better to retire early and arise early.

Drink 8-oz of distilled water long before you prepare for bed. Lie down with a smile on your face. Feel the smile. Think how you are becoming clean as you slip into a pleasant slumber.

Day Four

Arise early, admiring the beauty of daylight. Sit for 15 minutes in sunlight before dressing (if available). Sip a glass of distilled water upon arising. After your sunbath (in the nude whenever possible) drink, by chewing, your first glass of H.A.R.A.

Plan out some physical activity that you are attracted to. Remember "working out" is sometimes called "work" by persons *not* wellness oriented. Cutting the grass is "work" to some people, but to a body aware of its need to become clean, it is "work out!" The same is true of walking or biking, whether on an errand or "out for exercise."

Rest in the late morning, or in the early afternoon. Spend some "rest time" listening to soft music (jazz, classical, blues, country-Western, instrumental, seasonal or patriotic). Keep the volume low enough to be heard, but not loud enough to 'require' your attention.

An hour after music, meditate for 20 minutes. Smile with the pleasure that comes from becoming clean. Feel yourself smile. In the early evening, consider a number of personal acts or incidents that need your forgiveness.

Try to imagine how each time you forgive, a little more 'stored garbage' from your mind and body is being removed. Each time you forgive—or say, "I forgive," feel the cleansing taking place in your own body. Smile at the release from mental stress you feel occurring within you.

Reflect upon acts for which you wish to be forgiven. Line them all up. *Begin to receive forgiveness by forgiving yourself.* Say aloud: "I forgive myself for (whatever); and I forgive myself for...(whatever else).

Continue to forgive yourself until you have named each and every single deed or action, attitude or belief that you want to be forgiven for. Do not be concerned whether you are to be forgiven by the individual or individuals you offended. That will come later.

In the quiet time before bed, read some of your favorite poetry. If you have no favorite, read from what is available. If nothing else is handy, read some of the shorter Psalms. Do not try to figure out all the meaning; just read quietly and smile. Think to yourself: "I am becoming clean. It is working. What I am doing is working to get me clean."

Now, you can admit to yourself: "I am becoming happier. I am feeling better about myself. I am thankful for what is happening to me." Go to bed, about two hours after drinking one 8-oz glass of H.A.R.A for the evening.

Remember, it is okay to get up during the night to urinate or to move your bowels. Just return to bed, close your eyes, smile and clear your mind. Smile and return to your slumber. But, if you are one who cannot go back to sleep after getting up, perhaps you should drink nothing at least three hours before bedtime.

Day Five

Arise early. Drink a glass of distilled water. Move your bowels; and begin an animated work out. Go on for from 30 to 60 minutes. Begin your workout by stretching all the limbs and by flexing all the joints. End each workout by doing the same things as when you started.

Rest for a time after working out. Slowly "chew" down some H.A.R.A. (and/or distilled water, depending upon what your body 'tells' you it wants/needs). Learn to listen to your body. Practice *obeying* the messages, instructions, or "notions" you receive. Become comfortable trusting these messages your body/mind intelligence sends to you. "It takes a long time on raw foods and extra rest," says Dr. Vetrano, "to be able to trust your instincts."

After resting, do something creative: read, paint, sing, think. Keep yourself calm, and remain in a quiet, orderly environment. Think only of pleasant things. Consider no "problems," either your own or anybody else's.

Believe that the world is becoming cleaner, just as you, yourself, are becoming cleaner. And, be content and thankful that this cleansing process is happening.

See all the concerns you ever had about health, or sickness or disease being cleaned away from you and from the larger world. See yourself as a representative of the whole world. Envision your body as the entire earth, and your mind as the "heavens above." See the cleansing going on in your own body also going on in the world about you. Say aloud to yourself: "Just as I am becoming cleaner so, too, is the world about me becoming cleaner." Smile and feel yourself smiling.

Rest. After resting, meditate for about 20 minutes. Clear your mind of all "logical thoughts." If it helps, chant or hum, or whistle softly, taking deep breathes (inhaling and exhaling). Smile and feel yourself smiling.

Day Six

Upon arising take a half glass (4-oz) of H.A.R.A. If your body desires more fluid drink ("chew down") 4oz of distilled water. Within 30 minutes you should have your first bowel movement of the day.

If you have taken no food all these days (which is what I recommend)—no fruits, no fruit or vegetable juices, no other green vegetables, no nuts or seeds, and no less recommended foodstuff—you may not be inclined to as frequent bowel movements. This is normal.

Fill the bathtub with water, as hot as is comfortable for you and gently sit yourself into the water. Remain seated for so long as the water feels hot-to-very warm. 15 to 20 minutes should be sufficient. After drying yourself, dress warmly and comfortably; then, rest for at least one hour. Take care not to be in a draft, or to fall asleep while perspiring.

Repeat the Seitz bath every other day, or at least 4 times during the week. Unless vigorous exercise and frequent bowel movements have occurred, on the alternate days, do recommended physical exercises. At bedtime, meditate for 20 minutes. "See" how beautifully your body's cleansing is coming along. Tell yourself: "My mind is becoming cleaner. It is working. What I am doing is working to clean my mind; and, I am thankful." Drink a half glass of H.A.R.A. as you retire. Smile yourself to sleep.

Day Seven

Wake up early to a bright, new day—no matter what the weather, or the state of affairs in the world. Tune out any "current events" and listen to no news reports or commentaries on either radio or television. Avoid "talk shows" and their discussions. Do not listen to "religious broadcasts." Avoid loud music or other noises.

Have a glass of H.A.R.A. and think uplifting thoughts. Gaze into the glass of H.A.R.A. and imagine all those "planets in the universe." See all those "protective pawns" that will enter the universe of your body and make it clean and organized.

See yourself and your body as the foundation of the universe itself. Contemplate your mental processes as the 'Divine Mind' at work. Know, as you move slowly into your seventh day, that this has been time "Divine Wisdom" has used to create an entirely new universe, *an entirely new you.*

Rest for some 20 to 30 minutes, contemplating the cleaner condition of your insides. Imagine the purity of your mind. See the empty spaces in your body and in your mind, where once all sorts and manner of uncleanness once occupied. Give quiet thanks for the new, cleaner <u>you</u>.

Drink 8-0z of cranberry cocktail juice slowly while relaxing. Follow later with 8oz of distilled water. See the "muddy water" of your past being now all cleaned up. Give thanks, again. Smile. Feel yourself smiling. Be grateful. Feel yourself being grateful.

Meditate. Spend 20-30 minutes appreciating the new you. Look inside yourself, at your cleaned out body; at your cleaned out mind. Smile at what you see. Know in your heart that what you want has happened. You have become clean; and, you are very grateful. Express your gratitude to your "God." Listen to your own words. Feel your smiling gratitude.

Say to yourself: "I have become clean. What I did worked. My actions have made me clean. I am proud of myself. I am grateful that 'God' helped me have the strength, the determination, the will power, to clean up my body temple and my mind temple.

Rest now. Awaken or arising from rest, meditate. See the cleanliness of your insides. Know the purity you now enjoy. Anticipate the great feeling of wellness that is enveloping your entire organism.

Know that you can now contemplate, as you sip away on a glass of H.A.R.A. how you might serve others who will need to share your cleansing experiences.

Day Eight

Pray, meditate, be quiet all day; give thanks that you are alive, and **well on your way to an addiction-free lifestyle.**

Consider whether you want to repeat the program, starting at Day 2 and coming forward; or, starting on any given day. Consider how long you have been addicted to the substances that have controlled your life. Now, consider how short a time you have just spent "cleaning up."

Give yourself a fair chance to survive and overcome; make the right decision for yourself, for your situation. Repeat this entire program as many times as you feel inclined. However, if you have abstained from food these many days, re-read the Chapter on *Therapeutic Fasting*. Follow the instructions/suggestions given there—especially on **"How to End Your Fast."**

These are important companion Chapters. Permit them to serve you well.

Chapter Nine

Toward a Reliable Theory of Disease

The popular perception of disease is that it is "a bad omen" which affects innocent people: young people, fat people, skinny people, middle-aged people, sick people, old people; and, it is most sinister because it also "attacks innocent children."

Internationally, there is the 'common belief' that "disease is caused by the invasion of some foreign or alien element into the mind and/or the body." Exactly 'what' invades the organism ranges from "evil spirits, curses and bad omen" to germs, viruses and 'bugs.'

Either the disease happens because "an innocent victim" becomes 'possessed' or because 'guilty parties' are being punished—or, perhaps, because an unlucky person is "in the wrong place at the wrong time." This latter notion also covers person-to-person and person-to-animal contacts.

Fundamental Concepts

1. Logical thinking or empirical observation tells us that "the world is <u>not</u> a perfect place." From whatever angle one wants to view this statement, the final conclusion short of the illogic of religious belief—is that human kind experiences a world with many inconsistencies, some of which are regularly occurring in Nature. And, while 'inconsistencies' are not necessarily indices of 'imperfections', our premise is that even when we reduce all down to the relative capacity of

the human organism to perceive that which exists, we do so imperfectly.'

2. Given 'the world' as it is, one Supreme Law regulates its vastness and diversity. Not that it is so simple as our earlier notion that "what goes up must come down." This law is one of relationship, a "duality of imperfection." An example of what this means might be put this way: (a) If you do not eat watermelon seeds, you will never find them in your stool. (b) A person who never flies in a commercial airliner will never become a disaster passenger of a commercial airline 'accident.' (c) One who never encounters a swimming pool will never drown in one. We could go on and on.

But, what is the point? The point, simply, is that the relationship we have been looking at is often referred to as 'cause and effect.' And, while we might argue its absolute domain, in reality, as we have hinted elsewhere, a relationship exists between what has happened (at any given time) and what will happen (at any present/future time).

3. 'Imperfection' is evident when inconsistencies show up. While cigarettes (tobacco products) cause 'cancer' and premature death, not everyone who uses these products comes down with cancer, or seems to suffer any plausible reduction in longevity. Five people fall from the sky in a light plane, or go over a cliff in an automobile, or are hit by enemy fire in a combat zone—and only one of these lives. And, we ask, "Why?' and will generally answer our own question with a special reference to "God."
4. To restate the central point, and move on: (a) if you are not in the vehicle, when it crashes, you are not one of the victims; (b) if you never possess a lottery ticket, you never can 'win' the lottery prize; (c) not "being at the wrong place at the wrong time" does not mean that you absolutely will not be a 'victim.'

5. Our notion of The Supreme Law of the Universe, as has been stated, historically, by my teachers and therefore by me, is absolutely incorrect. What science has taught us about the Law of Cause and Effect is a fallacy: physics, if that is the law's origin, is fundamentally incorrect. This is what has been demonstrated in all of our examples, above; and, this 'challenge' to an old, accepted scientific notion must be given serious reconsideration. All so-called science that proceeds, without coming to terms with this basic misunderstanding will continue to lead mankind toward the end of existence as we know it.
6. False constructs (believing that "a virus" is more life-threatening than are medications and chemicals) over the past one hundred years (in particular) have led mankind into a 'scientific cul-de-sac.' One example is we poison our water to kill bacteria and "viruses" (which are already dead matter); and, in doing so we destroy ourselves. The food problem is the same; we pasteurize and medicate milk to destroy virulent organisms, while at the same time destroying its food value and our people's health.
7. A clear-cut scenario is over drawn in John Robbins' book, ***Diet for a New America,*** and other contemporary treatises on ozone layer, greenhouse effect, ocean pollution, irradiated foods, "unaffordable health care" and on and on. The story of 'the hamburger,' for example, if followed out to its logical conclusion would lead to the final destruction of life as we know it, indeed to the extinction of the human race! ***Even vegetarians who survived the carnage brought on by the meat-consumption-cycle would, themselves, be finally cannibalized by carnivorous fellow humans.*** The "end" could come for all.

Reliable Concepts

1. The Supreme Law of the Universe, the one 'Law' that governs all—without exception—is:

(a) For every effect, there is at least one cause.

(1) Thus, the proper law upon which 'science' can rely is **The Law of Effects of Cause.**

(2) Perhaps more times than not, there are multiple "causes" that might be uncovered, once an effect is known.

(3) Investigations (criminal and tort) employ a scientific procedure that has been presumed of science itself.

(4) Perhaps, science's backward approach (reliance) is what "glorifies" 'extensive research, animal mutilations, environmental destruction, massive capital expenditures and wholesale public disappointment, ignorance, and despair.

(5) Often has this writer suggested that the scientific community (medical research) does not produce "a cure" for whatever "disease" because they are looking for the wrong thing in the wrong places and you cannot find rabbits at the tops of standing trees!

2. Disease when it is "an effect" surely has at least one (discoverable) cause. For the most part, this cause or these causes are ascertainable.

a. Applying the universal (as opposed to "scientific") principle of "effects of cause," does not imply that even if cause or causes can be known, "cure" or reversal, or a "healing" will be manipulated.

b. The "fundamental absolute" is that we must cease to conduct our affairs in such manners that will ultimately lead to our demise.

3. Disease, as the term is generally used, is always an "effect;" *it is never a "cause."* In fact, it could be an "interim effect;" or it could be a "terminal effect." As a ***mind/body cleansing process***, dis-ease is either interim or terminal, depending upon its long-term causes, compounded "causes," and/or "resultant causes." For example, long term alcohol consumption first impedes body function, then

diminishes affected body organs, and drugging, cutting and/or burning exacerbate these circumstances.

a. Disease may also produce a "genetic affect." A pot-smoking or cocaine father will likely give birth to a child with visible "handicaps." Sometimes, the "conditions" are not readily observable. They are potentially there, nonetheless, because at least our "cause" is readily knowable.

b. Again, what is being illustrated is <u>not</u> that there is a reliable "cause and effect" relationship between the mother (or father!) using drugs (any kind of drugs, incidentally!), but rather that when an effect (abnormality) is observed in the child there is now a perfect duality of relationship: where effect is visible, at least one cause ***must be*** parental consumption of drugs (medications, chemicals, toxins). ***As hard as this might be to swallow—parents—when your child is born with any 'handicap,' look to causation in your own consumptive lifestyles!***

c. Still out front as the most dangerous "legal drug," alcohol (beer, wine, spirits, and "coolers") is now outpacing prescription and over-the-counter drugs as the next biggest prenatal killer of American babies. Pharmaceuticals and chemicals, in this country, seem to have overtaken tobacco products, and are perhaps, the number-two health menace to babies in the United States.

d. How it all seems to work is this way: (a) Parents consume poisons (sleeping pills, for example!) that reduce the level of their body/mind functions and retard the performance of their vital body organs (or in the case of the male, for example, wipes out "essential chromosomes"). The results: a child is likely to be born that did not fully (normally) develop. Nor are grandparents <u>ever</u> to blame!

e. The "skip generation principle" cannot happen because it violates the absolute law: that where there is observable effect, there is discernible cause. In other words, a child born of a midget can produce a "normal" child. More precisely, however, a child with leukemia will, if it grows to maturity, produce either a non-leukemia child or no child at all. Of course, we mean to exempt this child from the same abusive lifestyle as was lived by its parent/s.

f. The above is not intended to send parents with handicapped children "on a guilt trip." It is, instead, aimed at helping such parents understand the connection between their babies' conditions and behaviors in our society that are considered either "legal" or all right! In this manner—and perhaps only then—future unborn generations can be spared the awful burden of providing careers, specializations and "vulgar incomes" to an entire network of "special interests" who perpetuate misinformation and feed on "common belief structures" (programmed ignorance). Are you acquainted with the term, "Special Education?"

g. Nor can this pen be stilled because powerful industries might perceive a threat to their incomes. Surely, many people reading this will change what they do; what they believe; and what they spend their money on. More importantly, however, the implications inherent in this presentation could stare humankind away from self-destruction. Besides, even if it were generally known—and substantially believed (that consuming certain things cause deformed births and premature deaths), people would continue, in large numbers to:

(1) Drink milk and eat dairy products.

(2) Drink beer, wine, and other spirits.

(3) Consume over-the-counter, prescription, and 'recreational' drugs and chemical substances.

(4) Eat hamburgers and other meats as a food staple.

(5) Drink "soft drinks," artificial juice drinks, and other sugar-dependent beverages.

(6) Use tobacco products and also overdose on animal protein consumption; and these are things individuals do to themselves.

(7) Being poisoned by participation in military campaigns, or from city water supplies, or from air pollution, or food growing and marketing, or from everything from indoor toxins to workplace health hazards, and ordinary household chemicals is, in a real sense, "civigenics" (poisoning at the hands of others)! What all this means, therefore, is that would-be parents do not do what is best for their unborn children (just as they do not do what is best for themselves!) simply because they know and accept what is untrue information. Therefore, "Wall Street" is safe; and people do take the option of "committing suicide," even when they decline to prevent homicide or genocide.

"But, What Can I Do?"

1. Direct action requires a purpose or motive or objective. When there is one in place, course or courses of action are much clearer. For example, a drinking person who wants to become a parent will cease all known debilitating consumptive behaviors; such parents will stop drinking alcohol, soft drinks, coffee, tea, and so forth.

2. That individual will see to it that the perspective mate does the same thing.

3. Allow a suitable period of time for the organism to cleanse or rid itself of retained toxins.

4. Guarantee the unborn the "right" to pass into this life free from handicaps based solely upon parental consumptive lifestyles.

Summary

What has been presented here might be provocative. That in itself is potentially useful. Sentiments notwithstanding, the following are statements to be given thoughtful consideration:

1. Where there is a visible or known condition ("effect"), you can reasonably search out the cause or causes.

2. Sickness, disease, and premature death are "effects." Less than the terminal effect of death allows a possible opportunity to remove the "causes."

3. The Law of "Effects of Cause" is totally redemptive for the human race.

4. Wellness, in any time or culture—ultimately—is taken seriously and implemented only by "people who care about wellness."

5. Massive changes in public consumption patterns—from that which reduces wellness to that which improves wellness—will preserve individual and plant healthfulness, but will not put out of business those who make markets in "stuff" not good for human consumption.

The reason the "fast food" industry, for example, will thrive is, given what we all know about human behavior, we are very aware of the tendency for people to do what they enjoy as opposed to what is best for them—even when they know the difference! People learn to do and prefer what feels good and what tastes good. Sugar is the "goddess" of taste.

Chapter Ten

Some Salient Physiological Principles (T. C. Fry's own [last] words)

Herbs, Drugs, Modalities, and Human Traits. As you conclude your first reading of ***The Nature and Purpose of Disease,*** I feel it appropriate to remind the reader of some of the salient physiological principles presented, directly and indirectly, in this book.

1. That which stimulates or occasions an action is the offending substance against which the action is directed.

2. Cancer cells do not invade the body. They are the body's own cells that seceded from the body autonomy because of inimical substances including oxygen deprivation that not only seriously deranged them but also threatened their existence.

3. Lecithin, to the extent required, is synthesized by body faculties, particularly the liver, from organic phosphorus and fatty acids. Alien lecithin is unusable and must first be digested and assimilated before being synthesized according to the body's own unique pattern.

4. The idea of loading the body with more than it can use is nutrient-gluttony. The body can safely handle endogenous overproduction and even ingested excesses of futile nutrients. However, synthetic and other indigestible substances cannot be used and are ejected at great expense to body faculties and energies.

5. Crutches cripple! We lost our ability to synthesize vitamin C back in antiquity when nature created a food package around seeds to induce our consumption with the incidental benefit of having us distribute their seeds. Uncannily, the products that were created to induce our symbiotic cooperation met our nutrient needs so well that it was no longer necessary for the body to synthesize many nutrients, vitamin C included.

When you do not use a faculty you lose it! Unused faculties atrophy. Usage develops and strengthens faculties.

If you cease to use one leg by using crutches, compensatory usage falls on the other leg, the shoulders and the arms. The unused leg withers. The extraordinarily used arms, shoulders, and leg become larger and more muscled.

The use of insulin from extraneous sources tends to cause atrophy of the beta cells of the Isles of Langerhans in the pancreas. Thus, in about three to four years, even a perfectly healthy pancreas will probably lose its ability to synthesize insulin!

Thus, the intake of other body nutrients directly into the body economy or their ingestion tends to relieve the body of the secretary task! The body becomes dependent on the outside supply. Again, unused faculties atrophy and often, beyond redemption.

6. Herbs cure nothing! To say they do is to impute to them powers and intelligence they do not possess. To help the body as they purportedly do, they must know human physiology well enough to know what to do and have the physiological know-how to substitute for body wisdom, faculties, and resources.

Of course, only the body has the faculties, the resources, the intelligence, and the power to recognize oneself and inimical substances, to apprehend, seize and expel them from the vital domain. Only the body has the ability to recreate and replace injured cells and tissues. This is an innate ability of all organisms and cannot be done for the body by exogenous agencies called medicines or herbs.

Herbs do occasion body actions! As set forth in entry one herein before, the action begotten is directed against the unwelcome substances which occasioned the action. This brings us to another phenomena, that of overcompensation.

7. How the body overcompensates to insure benefits! It is well—established that vigorous exercise begets an extraordinary development of musculature and faculties to cope with the tasks undertaken. Up to a point, the development is beyond the requirements of the task; the body seeks to perform all tasks with facility and ease.

Vigorous aerobic exercises double and triple the metabolic rate of the body, thus creating wastes extraordinary to the norm. Likewise the body's eliminative faculties double and triple their function as well. Further, while in the eliminative mode, the heightened functions not only eliminate the extraordinary wastes generated, but overcompensate in that they also eliminate wastes and toxic matters that were theretofore accumulating in the vital domain.

The same principle applies to herbs and drugs when ingested or injected. The body turns on the alarms and goes into a frenzy of extraordinary elimination to expel the offending obnoxious and life-sapping poisons that inhere in the drugs or herbs. Upon the ingestion or injection of herbs and drugs, other eliminative tasks such as those involved in illnesses are deferred or discontinued until the worse enemy within is dealt with. This resulting cessation/deferral is called drug or herbal suppression of symptoms, which is almost universally mistaken for healing even though, in fact, the body is worse off. The original toxic load remains and the devitalizing drugs or herbs additionally assault body faculties.

However, the body may go into such an intense emergency that it not only eliminates the alien poisons ingested or injected but overcompensates and eliminates other toxic accumulations as well.

The result is usually exhaustion of the nerve energy required to conduct the emergency crisis. As a result the herb or drug taker suffers a hangover or what are better known as withdrawal symptoms.

Drug withdrawal symptoms are usually so severe that the drug taker is impelled to ingest or inject these or other drugs anew, thus again quelling the body's vital efforts again and begetting the 'high' feelings born of the body's frenzied attempts at extraordinary elimination.

Of such successive bouts are born addictions to poisons as contained in foods, herbs, and drugs.

8. Substances that stimulate or heighten a function above normal also depress and lower that function. Those who ingest caffeine or its cousins theine and theobromine as found in coffee, soft drinks, chocolates, and teas experience heightened mental powers. As a concomitant of the emergency eliminative mode the body enters into, and to deal with life-sapping substances, it secretes noradrenaline or norepinephrine and even endorphins to spur body operations and mask the pain. These are the substances that beget the 'high' experienced when poisons are ingested. The result is exhaustion of faculties and subsequent withdrawal symptoms which, when quelled with new dosages, becomes fixed as an addiction.

9. Disease is not an entity. The only initiative quality is the body, which conducts processes that manifest as disease. What are called diseases are the symptoms of an overwhelmed body dealing with a life-threatening load of accumulated toxic materials.

Suppressing body efforts with drug poisons as in herbs and drugs is a process of debilitation that makes eliminative problems continuous or chronic.

10. Just as physical exercise develops physical fitness, so too does mental exercise develop mental fitness. Thus thinking, cogitation, and related mental activities develop mental fitness and acuity of a high order! The order is higher yet when mentation, whether in appropriating knowledge as in learning or in creativity as in writing, is accompanied by beauty in sound

(music), smell (fragrances) and sight (as in flowers, fruits, etc. which conduce to human well-being).

11. Stress is often not a case of what's wrong with you so much as who's wrong for you. When causes of problems are discontinued, removed, or avoided, the body no longer experiences the suffering that it did theretofore and sets about repairing the damages sustained.

12. The concept of medicine is erroneous. There can be no "curative" or healing substance, agency, or modality! All healing is exclusively and only self-healing. At best this can be facilitated in some cases such as suturing rent flesh or setting bones in place. That might power and intelligence which developed each of us from a microscopic fertilized ovum is the only power capable of assessing a body's problem and rectifying it. It's the only power capable of detoxifying the body, knitting bones, and creating new cells and new tissues.

13. Our study of nutrition has to do with our nutrient needs and how best to supply them for wonderful health, not the so-called Basic Four or really the Basic Five which is really a scheme to assure commercial interest a niche in the junk food marketplace, as Dr. Anderson points out in his hypothetical "convention on nutrition" in the Author's Preface.

14. Practically every fruit you can name has everything you need in about the exact proportion that your body requires it, that is, aside from water and fiber. Fruit solids contain 85% to 90% glucose and fructose, about 5% amino acids, about 3% minerals, about 2% fatty acids and about 1% vitamins and miscellaneous nutrients, largely uncharted food factors.

Fruits are predigested for humans when ripe. They are super delicious and at their nutrient peak. They have made themselves into a dietary delight to attract consumption by their biological symbiont.

15. Fair warning! While there are lots of calories in starchy foods such as legumes, grains, roots, and tubers there is an unforgivable evil involved in their consumption: cooking. Cooking deranges their wealth of nutrients, especially protein,

and quite literally leaves proteins a pathogenic mess. Heating proteins above 150 degrees Fahrenheit renders them unusable by the body. They have been deanimated.

Heated proteins are soil for putrefaction in the intestinal tract by bacterial and fungal flora which will yield a plethora of poisons like hydrogen sulfide, indole, skatole, mercaptans, ammonia, putrescence, cadaverine, and so on, all quite pathogenic and carcinogenic.

Heated fats, which are substantial in legumes, especially in soybeans and tofu, are quite pathogenic and carcinogenic. According to the Food and Drug Administration's Office of Toxicological Sciences, cooked meats, including fish and chicken, contain a heat-created by-product called nitrophyrene. It is toxic and carcinogenic. When you heat tofu and beans (globulin), you not only get nitropyrene but yet another carcinogen: indole. (Also refer to the book published by the National Research Council of the National Academy of Sciences in 1982 titled: Diet, Nutrition, and Cancer).

16. Highly vaunted alfalfa sprouts, which are a current craze, contain a substance, canavanine, which we, unlike horses and other animals, secrete no enzyme to break down.

17. I eat what I like most or that makes me feel the best. I love eating mostly all-dessert meals. I am—as are you—a fruitarian, by Nature's preference!

"My children are killed for lack of knowledge," says the god of the Hebrew scriptures. Millions die yearly because they lack true conceptions of life, of health, of disease, of cure. More people are killed every year by the cause of and the treatment for "disease" than by any other causes, only because their ignorance leads them to ignore causes and to rely upon "cures."

- *T.C. Fry (1974)*

Chapter Eleven

'Garbage-In Equals Garbage-Out'

Many pages and a lot of words have been used to say something so very simple: what is consumed—physiologically and psychologically—guarantees, for the most part, whether one experiences good health, happiness, and long life or an abbreviated life, characterized by sickness, disease and a resultant lower quality of living.

With encouragement and support from Dr. T. C. Fry, my most respected mentor and Natural Hygiene guru, the fruitarian "do the right thing" message has been presented from a metaphysical standpoint, a common sense perspective, the "scientific view," from confirmation by personal experience, and by many references to respected researchers who have no particular interest in these representations.

Some principles, heretofore considered 'absolutes,' may now look differently to you. Perhaps, it is troubling that what has been presented and taught, as the law of "cause and effect" is, quite simply, the Law of "Effects and Cause." These rollover "effects," in turn are perceived as 'new causes.' For, we know now that good health is no accident!

Dr. Fry has expressed it so succinctly: "Diseases cannot be prevented while their causes are in force. Diseases do not have to be prevented inasmuch as they will not happen unless caused."

Many people understand this rule; some do not. Many people will never know these truths; some will know but will not care. Many people will continue to suffer sickness and disease—even if reliable information is available; some will live sickness and disease free. Whether lives are lived in ignorance, or in full knowledge—of these or other principles—consumptive behaviors will still determine quality of life; and, as we all know, aside from 'quality of life,' ***none of us will get out of this rat race alive!***

Above all, know this: behaviors that result in the onset of disease symptoms must be discontinued, if one wishes to avoid or prevent the eventuality of sickness and disease. *'Prevention,' then, is the only 'cure' worthy of reliance.*

Preventing sickness and disease—while the most essential safe guard for 'quality of life' preservation—is not entirely within the control of the individual. Nonetheless, using or maximizing the predominant control we can have will offer the best assurance of a healthy, happy quality of life.

Three principle regimens are explored and are offered as appropriate vital strategies for an individually managed wellness program. These are (1) fasting regularly (at least every three-to-six months); (2) natural or unassisted elimination (one to four times daily, without force, laxative, or other than organically fibrous foods intake; and (3) exercising and stretching all the joints in the body at least three times weekly (working up a sweat and requiring a period of rest afterwards). Without these three it is doubtful one can effect the maximum prevention against occasional sickness and/or cumulative dis-ease in the organism.

Finally this: in the modern would, toxic/carcinogenic factors are so pervasive, there are two clear options: (1) choose a fruitarian, hygienic, and organic consumption lifestyle, or (2) continue to gain weight, for it is in the fatty tissues the body is better able to distract toxic carcinogenic agents away from the blood stream, thereby forestalling the organism's demise for some additional time.

But, this discussion cannot conclude without specific attention to understanding _the nature of disease_ when children are the subjects of a wide variety of disease symptoms. This reflection is important for two reasons: (1) We have shown, by actual reference and by implication, that "the diseases" about which society is most preoccupied in later life begin in childhood; and (2) Young children are totally dependent upon adult caretakers to provide for them what is best for them; and adults—especially parents—are most vulnerable: responsible to the children, to society, and to themselves, pretty much in that order.

Diseases and 'Myths' in Infancy

Children are born into the world with the best their biological parents could offer. In most cases, that offering is adequate. But, in many instances, it is not. Mothers and/or fathers who smoke, eat chocolates, indulge in cooked foods, take medications, consume alcohol, or use other types of drugs might give birth to children with a variety of "birth defects," including but not limited to "HIV."

The literature is replete with evidence that fathers who were exposed to Agent Orange in Vietnam, and those who fought in the Gulf War witness neurological and other deformities in their offspring. Very often beer drinkers and "fast food fathers" are told their children's birth defects "are genetic," implying what has befallen the children bears no relationship to the consumptive behaviors of the parent/s. Of course, this notion is palatable and relieves guilt or 'responsibility;' but it is pure 'myth.'

A child cannot have better substance than the parents can give; nor, for that matter, is a child likely to exhibit defects unless the 'causes' are present in the bodies of the parents. A child born a midget, for example, because the mother—or father—took "designer drugs" as were popular during their 'youthful years' will sire a 'normal' child, provided similar destructive behaviors are not engaged.

A child born with leukemia, or Lupus, or muscular dystrophy, or whatever, is a reflection of the internal contents of the parents who birthed that child. Health begets health. Toxemia begets toxemia. This is why tumors removed by surgery very often reoccur. The natural law of 'cause and effect' is operative, not for the poor and uneducated, but for the rich and educated as well. Causes produce effects. Disease symptoms are, as we have shown over and over, 'effects.'

Etiology of Diseases in Children

In the United States of America, nearly 40% of all children die of cancer, according to Dr. T. C. Fry and others. Yet, despite this despicable statistic, parents, and grandparents still corral children and haul them off to "cute eating places," the McDonald and the Chuck E. Cheese and the Domino Pizza, as examples, setting them up for the onset of cancerous cells over time. This 'McDonald-Domino Syndrome,' is perhaps the best way to describe how the SAD (Standard American Diet) conspires to kill off our children right before our eyes!

In 'defense of' the fast food industry, children's demise begins long before they are able to 'appreciate' the clown and cartoon characters and other marketing gimmicks used to lure old and young alike into fast food establishments. Mothers begin with their own milk, when they have not prepared their bodies with healthful habits. Thus, the 'immunity' promised in mother's milk is not always realized by the infant.

Next, children are fed cereals and other starches long before teething, when their small bodies have not produced the metabolic enzyme necessary to break down starch. So, the stuff is retained in the child's system, only to ferment and putrefy. No wonder small babies have such foul stools when they are not raised on live foods!

Very early on, instead of fresh made juices from organic fruits and vegetables, children are fed cow's milk (which some researchers report might contain up to 200 or more drugs and chemicals, including antibiotics and pesticides). What's more, this cow's milk, which is purchased from the local supermarket and fed to babies is so lethal, if fed back to the cows, says the late Dr. Alvenia M. Fulton of Chicago, would cause instant death! Milk and diary products do not "build strong bodies or strong bones," as the public is told, but rather build mucus and acidity, ideal environments for the growth and multiplication of bacteria within the infant body.

If this is true, "Why doesn't the government stop it?" you ask. Anne E. Frahm, who overcame "terminal cancer which had metastasized to her bones," answers thusly: "Milk is the most political food in the United States...our taxes go to underwrite the dairy industry 'to the tune of almost three billion dollars a year... $342,000 every hour...The government buys dairy surplus to keep production going, letting it rot in storage at a cost $47 million annually. Millions more are spent by the National Dairy Council every year to get us to drink their product and help reduce their huge surplus...."

"What's even more critical according to Harvey Diamond," Frahm writes, "is that "people are consuming dairy products for calcium, and the existing calcium in their systems is being used to neutralize the effects of the dairy products they are eating...All dairy products for butter are extremely acid-forming." Diamond refers to milk and dairy product consumption as "taking two steps forward and three back."

The Acid-Alkaline Balance in Children

The very best foods humans can consume are fruits, vegetables, nuts, and seeds raw and organically grown. What is "true for the goose is true for the gander." There is no better source of calcium, protein, minerals, non-cholesterol fats, vitamins, and minerals than through the foods the human organism is anatomically created to consume. These foods are best for children of all ages, from infancy to very old age.

Children who consume SAD often suffer from 'over-acidity.' Under such conditions, fermentation produces vinegar and alcohol, soil for bacterial decomposition in babies' stomachs. Add our preoccupation with feeding children candy and sweets and the stage is set for sickness and disease from the earliest years of these young lives. Ever wonder why our children are so "out of control?" Just look at what they consume, by way of diet and entertainment! Cooked, deranged foods are their stable; and murder and violence are 'the art forms,' the essential ingredients, along with sex, in American drama and "video games."

Children's physiology is out of balance, from their diets and from excitement in their lives. ***John H. Tilden, M.D. says these lead to enervation, and enervation is the forerunner of toxemia; and, toxemia is the basic cause of disease.*** Yes, what we refer to as "diseases" are the effects of toxemia—cause.

Like the adults from whom they are conditioned, children are emotional and they harbor fears. *Fear and worry—mental devastation—kill more than 90% of the adults diagnosed with "terminal diseases."* Children also 'worry themselves to death' and set up internal conditions that give rise to the onset of degenerative disease conditions, sometimes with such intensity the child's life is spent before the adult world is aware of the crisis.

Vaccinations, Inoculations, and Immunity

Perhaps the second most lethal invasion into the fragile systems of children is the culture of so-called 'immunity injections' forced upon them by the same agencies of government which earlier persuaded parents to feed their babies cows' milk. Going back to 1872, Dr. Herbert M. Shelton found that *the largest number of smallpox deaths occurred when the largest number of babies was vaccinated 'to prevent the disease.'*

Deaths occurred from "serum poisoning" then as it does now, contrary to ***"the absurd medical notion that certain inoculated diseases confer immunity to future attacks***. There is not an iota of evidence in favor of this ancient superstition and every physician should know this. Yet they all subscribe to it in the case of a few diseases, although they freely confess that most of the 'injections' do not confer immunity. The whole of the vaccine and serum practice is based on this insane notion."

When parents ask, "What can I do to raise healthy children?" The answer is too simple, so simple in fact no matter how many times it is stated, or in how many ways, it goes unheeded because of the challenge to overcome earlier learning. So, permit me to respond in this manner: There are children—hundreds and thousands living in the United States of America who have never been sick, have no cavities, wear no eye glasses, are quite fit and are extremely intelligent. Likewise, these children have never eaten a hot dog, or tasted a 'soft drink,' nor have they been vaccinated or consumed cow's milk!

Chapter Twelve

"Interview with T. C. Fry"

This "Interview" with T.C. Fry occurred between September 18, 1999 and September 30, 1999, in Ikeja, Lagos [Nigeria], West Africa. © 1999 by Henry L. N. Anderson, Ed.D., Fruitarian and Protégé of Dr. Fry).

ANDERSON: Mr. Fry, before beginning this 'interview,' I would like to state some facts about you. **One**, you really are **Dr. T. C. Fry**, having been awarded an honorary Doctor of Science degree from City University Los Angeles in 1986, I believe.

Two, you wrote, among other publications, the book, ***The Great AIDS Hoax*** (Life Science Institute, 1989, ISBN# 1-55830-005-8). **Three**, you became a disciple of Dr. Herbert M. Shelton around 1970. **Four**, you wrote and published other books, newsletters, magazines, articles and portions of books authored by others. **Five**, your "Life Science Course of study" was adopted and is used in the curriculum of a medical school in France. **Six**, you changed many lives by your admonition people should not poison themselves, that "Only three substances should ever enter the human body! These are, obviously, good air, pure water and foods to which we are biologically adapted." [***Hoax***, p. 48, Item #23] **Seven**, you were the acknowledged mentor to Harvey and Marilyn Diamond, co-authors of the best seller, ***Fit for Life***. **Eight**, you contributed original pieces to this Volume and made other written and verbal contributions to the author as well. **Nine,** and finally, **you died on Friday, September 6, 1996, some time after returning to the U.S. with a friend from "an ozone treatment facility in the Dominican Republic run by a German," where your friend 'experimented' by taking one treatment while you "took about ten ozone treatments altogether."**

Now, some three years and three weeks **after your death** I conduct this 'interview' so that our readers—some of them new—can get to know you better. Your responses will not only be re-printed just as your words are written, but on each occasion, your particular reference will be cited so that anyone may review your fuller statements and/or verify your points of view.

Let me begin, then, with this observation and question: Most of us do not have access to electronic and print media; we can't even protect our children from the army of marketing people who lure them into their 'disease nets' with candy displays, fast food play lands, special birthday parties, and so-called "protective vaccinations." **What can parents do?**

T. C. FRY: Some tragic and starling revelations are surfacing about a new vaccine the drug establishment is pushing. The vaccine, called Hib for Hoemophilus Influenza type b, is administered to "prevent meningitis."

Meningitis is an inflammation of the membranes that cover the spine and brain. Irritating toxic substances occasions inflammation. In response the body creates a fever to intensity efforts to deal with these substances which are usually ingested and absorbed from the intestinal tract. When these permeate certain tissues, the body undertakes defensive reactions, such as fevers, to facilitate and accelerate their elimination.

Meningitis is said to kill about one thousand children annually in the U.S.A.

A large controversy is brewing about the use of this newly introduced vaccine. In certain states, Minnesota being the main one, more children are developing meningitis and dying of the vaccine than were affected before its introduction!

ANDERSON: You seem to be suggesting that parents are, somehow, 'led' into believing what is not true, and are, therefore, taken advantage of –by whom?

FRY: Let us review **the hoaxes** frequently foisted upon our people. In the late 1940s a new disease was foisted upon the American people. It was called polio. Several then-current diseases were renamed as polio. Among them were infantile paralysis, viral meningitis and aseptic meningitis. A hysteria and panic was created amongst our populace as was done in the case of what is called AIDS, and also a lumping together of several diseases, some of which have been in medical literature for well over one hundred years.

After the panic was build into a furor and an orchestrated hysterical demand for a vaccine that would prevent the problem, lo and behold, along comes Dr. Salk who developed a vaccine that would wipe out polio. And it did!

Simultaneous to the introduction of the vaccine the Centers for Disease Control introduced new diagnostic guidelines that relegated what would have been polio diagnoses back to the meningitis of pre-polio days. Only infantile paralysis remained as polio.

However, Dr. Salk's vaccine was quickly dropped, for it caused up to ten times the "polio" in those receiving the shots than was occurring in the unvaccinated. While Dr. Salk remained a hero despite the disastrous failure, the Sabine oral vaccine was quietly substituted in its stead.

ANDERSON: What could possibly be the motivation for so dastardly a deed?

FRY: The object of this commercial game is to market drugs, vaccines or whatever by creating a panic or hysteria around a "new" disease and then getting the populace to buy this drug forever after lest they contract the disease. As you can see the restitution of the diseases' original names effectively "wipes them out."

ANDERSON: You are saying, in effect, that parents cannot trust what they are being told. Is that what you would say to parents?

FRY: It is doubtful if even one thousand children per year were dying of meningitis. They, like so-called AIDS victims, are drugged and dosed with highly toxic drugs when they become sick. That these drugs do kill is self-evident for, when physicians go on strike, death rates plummet by up to 60%!

Our message is: Do not get caught up in these commercial voodoo games. They are deadly as well as costly. Healthful living always produces health. Vaccines and drugs are always disease producing and deadly. When your child becomes ill, a little fasting and a nontoxic diet of raw fruits, vegetables, nuts and seeds will restore high-level health.

There is no need for your child to suffer or die at the hands of a voodoo commercial monster with a voracious appetite for your dollars. [***The Great AIDS Hoax*,** pp. 135-136]

ANDERSON: People tend to 'know' wellness principles but do not implement those principles into their lifestyles, thereby preventing degenerative diseases from occurring in the first place. Why should people like you, Harvey Diamond, Dr. Ralph Cinque, Dr. Virginia Vetrano (M.D.), Prof. T. Colin Campbell, still others and me concern ourselves by all our pontificating about 'rules of wellness?'

FRY: ...Most people die in their ignorance, refusing to do better even if they know better. What do you think of a heavy smoker who after an operation for throat cancer, had a special device attached through an opening in his throat so he could continue his deadly addiction? [***Helping Hand***, pp. 120-121, #85].

Wellness begets long life. The mode of living that begets wellness also immensely enhances the quality of life.

The shorter the life span as a rule, the more miserable it is. People who neglect health live lives with more suffering and illness. Hence, their lack of care gives rise to perpetual discomforts and ailments. More than 50 percent of Americans suffer from chronic ailments either because "they don't care" or because they don't know enough to care. [***HH***, pp. 120, #84]

ANDERSON: Since we know for sure that wrong lifestyle behaviors lead to the so-called 'health problems' people experience later in life, how can people be motivated to pursue behaviors that will protect them from cancer, heart disease, diabetes, stroke, high blood pressure, arthritis, osteoporosis, and the symptoms lumped into the category of so-called AIDS?

FRY: Would you believe that perfect, sickness-free health is natural and normal? That disease and suffering are abnormal, unnatural and unnecessary? That bounding vigor and robust fitness are easy and certain? That...

Just as an airplane will fly millions of miles without mishap when it is properly cared for, so too, will your body last for at least 150 happy, rewarding years without sickness or suffering if its needs are likewise always properly met?

Would you believe that you can overcome, once and for all time your illnesses and ailments? That, whether it be indigestion, mucus expectoration, colds, flu bouts, headaches, backaches or even such "incurable" problems as acne, allergy, arthritis, asthma, tinnitus, tumors, or whatever, this system enables you to overcome all by simply discontinuing and removing easily-recognized causes, and establishing conditions that rebuild and maintain health?

Would you believe that there is a 100% effective health system?...I know this seems far out within the context of today's thinking and experiences. Ailments and illnesses, and discomforts and suffering are commonplace. But I want to assure you of one thing: You don't have to believe this! A totally effective health system is with us! It's called Natural Hygiene. [***HH***, pp. 1-2]

ANDERSON: People are stampeded by the notion of 'killer disease' because they do not want to die prematurely. Can people look to "cures" for their salvation?

FRY: Space permits only a very simple response to this question. The answer is No! There are NO CURES WHATSOEVER FROM ANY SOURCE!

An ailing or diseased body requires healing—physiological correction! All healing is a biological process AND ONLY THE AFFECTED ORGANISM HAS IN IT THE POWER TO HEAL! There are no other healing powers. The capacity to heal is inherent in the organism.

Diseases are symptoms of bodily healing crises. They are an evidence of vital action to expel morbid matters and to restore normal function.

ANDERSON: So, you dismiss all claims of "curing" made for all drugs?

FRY: Drugs furnish no nutrients. They have no intelligence to create new cells and repair damaged tissue. Instead drugs form chemical unions that paralyze nerves and suspend vital action, thus suppressing symptoms of disease. The person thus treated is sicker than before even though appearing and feeling better!

Drugs, which have a stimulant action rather than a narcotic action, goad the body into extraordinary eliminative activity but this exhausts an already exhausted body thus resulting in the subject being worse off than before.

ANDERSON: Many believe they are kept well and/or healed by their prescribed drugs. Are you saying they suffer an illusion?

FRY: All healing that takes place after the administration of drugs (or any other kind of treatment) does so in spite of the drugs, not because of them. Drugs and treatments all rise to glory on the back of the self-healing powers of the body!

Under no circumstances can drugs cure anything and there never will be such a drug. All drugs are inherently poisonous and dangerous to the organism. NO DRUG OF ANY KIND should ever be introduced into the human organism.

ANDERSON: You know you will be criticized as being too 'radical?'

FRY: Perhaps this subject has never received more illuminating treatment than that given to it by Dr. Herbert M. Shelton...[***Program for Dynamic Health,*** pp. 107-108]

ANDERSON: Is the public so into 'denial,' or the hypnotic spell of "slight of hand magic" that they continue to believe what defies logic, or are they systematically kept confused by deliberate cartel-orchestrated media misinformation?

FRY: One of the most vicious and harmful myths cultivated and perpetuated by the medical system is the modern version of visitations by demons and evil spirits. The modern version calls the beasties germs and viruses and terms the visitations contagion.

That bacteria and fungi do not cause disease and at worst, secondarily complicate infections is easily demonstrable by medical admission. By use of such words as susceptibility, non-susceptibility, low resistance and high resistance of disease, causation relegates itself to what constitutes susceptibility. Thusly, germs are opportunistic bystanders as they always were.

The mere presence of so-called disease causing germs and the absence of the disease is prima-facie evidence they do not cause disease. And when we suffer disease said to be caused by certain germs, and they are absent, this is more confirmation germs do not cause disease.

ANDERSON: In tropical areas, people believe germs carried by the mosquito cause malaria and other sicknesses; in Western cultures, people believe that 'cold germs' are responsible for 'spreading the common cold.' What do you say?

FRY: Diseases other than degenerative ones such as cancer, arthritis, cardiovascular problems, diabetes, et cetera, are body conducted emergency crises of detoxification and healing. Germs, thusly, have nothing to do with it.

Thus, disease is not an entiative existence, which can be spread. Insects spread filth, toxic substances and parasites, not diseases.

That humans manifest similar diseases merely confirms a self-evident observation that thoroughly discredits the myth of contagion. [***HH***, pp. 111-112, #57]

ANDERSON: I believe people have a God-given right to 'commit suicide'—by smoking, by drinking, by taking drugs, by consuming desserts, animal carcasses, sea creatures, air creatures and other flesh creatures—so long as they ***make a responsible choice***. My question to you, Dr. Fry, is how can people make responsible choices—whether to live or whether to die—if they are denied the "right" to know the truth?

FRY: Natural Hygiene is a total way of life that is fundamentally in accord with our biological disposition. When we conduct our lives within the purview of modern society as much as possible, diligently respecting our physiological needs, we'll realize far-reaching benefits that seem nothing short of miraculous!

Natural Hygiene holds that you're *almost totally* responsible for your well being! I say 'almost' in respect for our lack of control of environmental poisoning of our air and water. After all, health is built and maintained only by healthful living practices. Healthful living consists of supplying yourself with good air, pure water, comfortable temperatures, a clean body, adequate sleep, sunshine and natural light, rest and relaxation, vigorous activity, play and recreation, foods of your biological adaptation and yet other essentials. No one else can breathe for you, eat for you, sleep for you, exercise for you—in short, only you can live your life! [***HH***, pp. 1-2]

ANDERSON: What is the real story about the so-called AIDS epidemic?

FRY: The National Cancer Institute (NCI) is a distinct part of ***this monstrous cabal***. It is up to its ears in perpetrating the AIDS panic along with the Centers for Disease Control, the National Institute of Health and many other government agencies that run interference for the drug establishment.

You'll probably never read about what NCI did, nor the results it achieved when it commissioned Dr. Peter Duesberg of the Department of Molecular Biology and Virus Laboratories of the University of California, Berkeley, to make an exhaustive study of the so-called AIDS virus and its effects on humans.

ANDERSON: I can't say that I have. What were the results? What was Dr. Duesberg commissioned to do in the first place?

FRY: Under grant number CA39915A-01 from NCI, Dr. Duesberg did research on what are called HIV or human immunodeficiency viruses. Dr. Duesberg did just that, but he bit the hand that fed him! Whoever heard of research being made that did not serve the objectives of those funding the research?

An old saying has it that he who pays the fiddler calls the tune. Dr. Duesberg made the research and published his findings in a duly scientific manner in a report titled "Retroviruses as Carcinogens and Pathogens: Expectations and Reality." Instead of adding fuel to the fire of the AIDS promotion campaign, Dr. Duesberg's researches removed the props from under the shaky structure of viruses causing any disease at all, much less a degenerative disease called AIDS! So what did NCI do with the fiddler's tune? It relegated the report to the closet, where all bad boys belong. Their duplicity totally ignores the research and continues to proclaim viruses as causative agents in AIDS.

ANDERSON: Are you saying Dr. Duesberg was funded to validate faulty HIV research?

FRY: Koch's postulates, self-evident propositions, say that if any agency causes a disease, then that agency must always be present during that disease. If it is not present, then that means that it does not cause the disease. On the same order, if an agency causes a disease, then the presence of that agency must always occasion the disease. If the agency is present and the disease does not manifest, then that too means it is not the causative factor in the disease.

In his report, Dr. Duesberg noted that over 50% of those suffering from so-called AIDS did not have what are called human immunodeficiency viruses. That disposes of the claim, in itself, that AIDS is caused by a virus. But even more damning is the ballyhooed prospect of about one and a half million Americans getting the disease because they are said to have or have had the virus. If the virus caused the disease, we would have one and a half million suffers from AIDS! As threats, real or implied, are the raw materials from which panics and hysterias are manufactured, medical apologists have invented the excuse of "dormancy" in order that a fancied Damocles sword or time bomb hangs over those who are said to have or have had the virus. [***Hoax***, pp. 58-60]

ANDERSON: Who is behind "the AIDS conspiracy" and why deceive the whole world?

FRY: ***The Centers for Disease Control (CDC) is the primary agency responsible for originating, perpetrating and perpetuating one of the most villainous and evil conspiracies ever concocted!***

(1) Officials of CDC deliberately and callously introduced in fearful and frightful terms, as a new disease with the acronym AIDS, a collection of immunodeficiency diseases that had long been in the medical literature!

(2) Officials of CDC knew all the time that the pattern of symptoms they elected to introduce as AIDS **was drug-caused** and had previously been called certain stages of syphilis, Kaposi's syndrome, lymphocytopenia, pheumocystis carinii pneumonia and numerous other diseases. This was the import of numerous statements made by Dr. Harold Jaffe and Dr. James Curran originally together in the Center for Prevention Services, the Sexually Transmitted Diseases division. Now [1988-89] they head a division under the Center for Infectious Diseases dealing specifically with AIDS.

(3) They knew that 100% of the homosexuals suffering from what they elected to call AIDS (Kaposi's sarcoma, lymphocytopenia, "opportunistic infections," pneumocystis carinii pneumonia and late-state syphilis) were on the drugs amyl and/or butyl nitrite. They knew these drugs were classed as immunosuppressant drugs sold out

from under regulation as "deodorants." They knew that a member of the pharmaceutical combine, Burroughs-Wellcome, produced these drugs, among others and they knew that other drugs were often involved too.

(4) They knew from the beginning of the conspiracy that the pattern of symptoms they chose to publicize under the catchall acronym AIDS was being called GRID (Gay Related Immunodeficiency Disease) for the purpose of throttling and derailing the gay rights movement. They elected to go with the acronym AIDS, for it had implications that could apply to the general population as well as accomplish objectives of destroying the gay rights movement.

(5) They discontinued mentioning early on that ***100% of sufferers of the pattern of symptoms they chose to call AIDS were on recreational drugs or medically administered immunosuppressive drugs*** such as antibiotics, conticosteriods (prednisone, ACTH), alien blood products, and numerous other immunodestructive drugs. In fact, they did not usually point their fingers at any of the several immunosuppressive drugs the homosexuals were taking except heroin, which was administered intravenously.

(6) They knew that numerous cases of the affection they labeled as AIDS previously existed in the U.S. among the heterosexual white and black communities of drug addicts. But they chose to introduce AIDS in a most horrendous fashion, citing Haitian homosexual heroin addicts, taking care to emphasize the deadly and highly contagious character of this "baffling" new disease. ***They characterized the diseases as having originated in Haiti when they knew better. It originated in CDC!***

(7) From the beginning Dr. Jaffe and Dr. Curran knew that no virus was involved in AIDS. ***They knew it was a drug-caused problem***. They knew it was not contagious, being peculiar to those who committed acts of self-depredation with drugs. They knew that the disease they labeled AIDS existed

among people with kidney transplants who received immunosuppressive drugs, among those who suffered sexual diseases who had received massive does of antibiotics, and among those who, having tumors, had received X-rays and chemotherapy (all immunosuppressive).

(8) They angled their propaganda from the beginning of the conspiracy to hint that a virus or some single infectious agency caused the disease when they knew it was caused by immunosuppressive drugs and products.

(9) Dr. Robert Gallo purportedly discovered the causative virus when, in fact, the so-called virus he "discovered" as HTLV (human T-cell lymphotrophic virus) was really a dusting off of a "virus" he and his colleagues at the National Cancer Institute had introduced in 1980 as HTLV (human T-cell leukemia virus).

Yet, with this backdrop, officials at CDC chose to serve their own bureaucratic interest, research interests and, most of all, their pharmaceutical masters in staking out new markets for them.

They devised the acronym AIDS knowing that the disease was neither contagious nor transmitted. They did this with malice and evil intentions aforethought!

Yes, AIDS is the product of a conspiracy. The evidence and the actions bespeak this and only this. [***The Great AIDS Hoax***, pp. 192-194]

ANDERSON: To the cartel, your pronouncements and book, ***The Great AIDS Hoax***, are 'heresies.' Are you concerned for your well being?

FRY: In America and many other countries, an all-powerful, multi-trillion-dollar cartel controls about all there is to control that is of significance. In this country that cartel owns and/or controls virtually all the newspapers and magazines, all the TV and radio media, owns the chemical and drug industries, controls our governments, both state and federal, controls the medical/hospital system and, I repeat, about everything else that assumes economic/political importance.

Principal always overrides principle. Hence it has been aptly said that might makes right.

ANDERSON: Are you 'admitting' that even in a democratic society, individuals who 'swim up stream,' challenging Establishment positions, are somehow 'expendable?'

FRY: The system can put anything over on us it wishes! It has the power and the resources to make us believe anything it wants us to believe to better exploit us for its greater power and profit.

In the manufactured AIDS panic, all the cartel members coalesced to fool and scare our populace until it was in a frenzy of fear. All this was done so that a few more billion dollars would accrue to the medical/drug/hospital/research/bureaucratic interests.

The scam has been successfully pulled off, unlike the swine flu farce, and, indeed, billions of dollars have flowed into the coffers of those interests. In addition, much power and "prestige" have been conferred upon those instrumental in perpetrating and perpetuating such a monstrous hoax.

ANDERSON: We have some great minds in this country, and great institutions — like Harvard, Yale, Stanford, Berkeley, and others. How could such a farce be put over on an entire society — world, actually?

FRY: The technique employed has been called the Hitlerian Big Life Technique. This technique says: "If you tell a lie big enough, tell it often enough and tell it long enough, people will accept it as gospel truth."

We see this as being precisely the case with deliberate concoction of AIDS from a complex of symptoms called by more than 20 other disease designations. [***The Great AIDS Hoax***, pp. 203]

ANDERSON: What 'protection' does the public have from such continuing deception, deliberate misinformation, programmed stampede, and financial rip-offs?

FRY: As to a peril and a plague, why not call sleeping pills a peril and a plague? Twice as many people are dying of them as are dying of so-called AIDS!

When you realize that AIDS is, a big farce invented and fostered, firstly, to destroy the gay rights movement and, secondly, to stake out huge new economic reserves for our pharmaceutical and chemical industries, then you begin to perceive the truth. The sleeping pill business is safely in hand. The drug promoters want to develop new business. Of course they are seconded by power-hungry bureaucrats, opportunistic researchers and institutions, and a medical system that stands to benefit greatly....

ANDERSON: Assuming that what you say is true, what can we do about AIDS now?

FRY: What must be done about AIDS now? You should inform yourself about the atrocious plot to foist a bunch of old diseases on us under the guise of a new label for the greater financial glory of its beneficiaries. And, of course, do not be taken in by its fears or ensnaring webs. [***The Great AIDS Hoax*****,** pp. 207-208]

ANDERSON: I know you became a follower of Dr. Herbert Shelton and a 'Natural Hygienist' in 1970. Do you still believe Natural Hygiene has (all) the answers for optimum wellness, health and quality of life for people in much of the world?

FRY: In late 1970 when I made my GREAT HEALTH DISCOVER in the form of DR. HERBERT M. SHELTON'S fine book, *SUPERIOR NUTRITION*, I was very conformistic in my living practices.

At that time eating was not, for me, for the sole function of nourishing the body. Gourmandizing was one of my hobbies! In pursuit of the pleasures of what I now realize was a perverted and depraved taste I ate indiscriminately as long as eating was a "taste delight" and I never stopped to think about the purpose of eating or the consequences that might result.

I discovered Dr. Shelton's fine book on a holiday in 1970 among some of the many books I had purchased nearly 16 years earlier... I read *SUPERIOR NUTRITION* completely on the day of its discovery. I reread it within a week, marking it liberally where I found its contents to be nothing less than revelations for me.

So inspiring and so very obviously true was this book, that from that day to this I have not:

- Partaken of meat, fish, eggs, milk or any other animal food.
- Used a particle of salt, pepper, spices, mustard, sauces, catsup or any other condiment.
- Eaten or partaken of breads, chocolates, candies, ice creams, pastries or any of hundreds of other concoctions that are popular.
- Drank of teas, coffees, alcoholics or any other beverage than pure distilled water!
- Taken any drugs, shots, pain killers, sleeping pills, aspirins, antacid pills or concoctions, medicines", (sic) or any other injurious substances.
- Eaten but very little cooked foods!

Subsequently I stopped using soaps (cleansing is a mechanical, not a chemical process!), toothpastes, deodorants, shampoos, shaving creams, skin cleaners, lotions and other cosmetics!

ANDERSON: Over what period of time did you transition from meat eating to the Natural Hygiene way of thinking and eating?

FRY: I undertook most of these radical changes in my life IN A SINGLE DAY! So heavily did the truths of Dr. Shelton's book weigh upon me! I had always regarded myself as a creature of truth and it was beholden upon me to follow its dictates *upon discovery!*

So astounded was my family by this revolutionary turnabout in my regimen they thought I had gone kooky! [***Program for Dynamic Health*****,** pp. 3-4]

ANDERSON: Perhaps I overstated the last question. What advice do you have for people struggling with 'health issues,' and for parents with children?

FRY: Most American physicians who practice pediatrics ignorantly prescribe cereals, starchy and other solid foods for infants when they are some two or three months old. Never was a greater dietetic error committed! *It is a crime against children to be fed starches before (teething).*

Babies do not secrete the starch-splitting enzyme, ptyalin, until after they have teeth! This enzyme is absent from their saliva until then. Starches should not be fed to babies and to do so before they are biologically ready for them is to seriously impair and injure their health! Without the enzyme ptyalin starches cannot be digested! In a baby's stomach starches become sour, that is, they ferment, form vinegars and alcohols. Starches become the soil for bacterial decomposition in baby's stomach rather than food it can utilize.

The forcing of foods into a baby which is (sic) physiologically unsuited to it begins a life of dietetic depravity and perversion, a life of disease, physical debility and suffering. Babies wisely spit out foods not suited to them. They balk, refuse to eat and then spit out unsuitable foods. Babies aren't contrary—they're guided by body intelligence born of instinct and body chemistry. Only under great protest will babies finally ingest the bestial "foods" prescribed for them and which are literally forced into them.

It is no wonder that babies cry, are cantankerous, have stomach pains, indigestion, colic, vomiting, fevers, colds, foul stools, etc. Their loving mothers are forcing upon them a diet regimen prescribed by an almost universally ignorant medical profession! Ill health is visited upon babies by those who seek, above all things, health for babies!

It is any wonder that, wrongly fed and wrongly guided that 58.6% of our children cannot pass a minimum physical test? That **cancer is the number one killer of our children?** (Emphasis added). That obesity is so common among children as to cause no alarm? That the average child has such bad teeth it is criminal? Mothers who love their children can find no better way to care for their children than hygienic care. The NHA (formerly the American Natural Hygiene Society, PO Box 30630, Tampa, FL 33630) publishes an excellent book by Dr. Herbert M. Shelton, *THE HYGIENIC CARE OF CHILDREN*, which should be MUST READING for all mothers and mothers-to-be. [***Program for Dynamic Health*,** pp. 83-84]

ANDERSON: And, what of adults?

FRY: The average American poisons himself from 20 to 40 times a day with recreational drugs like tobacco, alcohol, soft drinks, cooked foods, fried foods, condiments and a whole host of materials unfit for human consumption. Only good air, pure water and raw foods of our biological adaptation should ever enter our bodies. Everything else is pathogenic. [***The Great AIDS Hoax***, p. 213]

ANDERSON: To my knowledge, this is the first time, perhaps since William Shakespeare, that an 'interview' has taken place between **a deceased person** (yourself) and **a 'still disillusioned' person** (this writer). What would you say is most significant about this 'interview?' Or, what would you say is the single most important message that can come out of ***this 'conversation' between the living and the dead?***

FRY: We have a propensity for believing what the establishment wants us to believe, and they trade liberally upon the cultivated myth of contagion. This makes more customers for their drug/medical/hospital trades.

If you live healthfully, you never suffer disease! Hygienic children never suffer "the usual childhood diseases." Diseases must be caused and only unhealthful practices cause them. [***The Great AIDS Hoax***, p. 104]

ANDERSON: Since the larger part of our 'interview' took place in Nigeria, West Africa, what have you to say about early attempts to link AIDS to the African continent?

FRY: The most "AIDS virus-infected" people in the world haven't one case of AIDS (1988-89)! Dr. Duesberg further points out that, in Africa where populations range from 20% to 60% body positive for the so-called AIDS virus, not one case of AIDS has ever occurred.

So what is the big AIDS hysteria about? Why is the establishment so intent on promoting it?

ANDERSON: That should have been my question! Is it only about money, really?

FRY: The AIDS promotion, like the swine flu farce and other CDC-orchestrated medical swindles, is one more rip-off called a boondoggle in the case of the CDC and a profit producer for pharmaceutical/research/medical interests.

In 1987 the federal and state governments spent in excess of one billion dollars on AIDS. In 1988 the projected costs will exceed $10 billion! That is what the AIDS panic is all about—a drive to stampede the American people into the medical-hospital- pharmaceutical corral for big bucks. That is what it's all about, not about saving people from diseases renamed and promoted under the fearsome banner AIDS. [***Hoax***, pp. 60-61]

ANDERSON: Does the medical establishment, which is controlled by the pharmaceutical/chemical cartel, use ethnicity and "any means necessary" to regularly prescribe drugs for humans and animals, knowing drugs are all toxic, because if they don't prescribe drugs and follow other establishment dictates they will not be permitted "to practice medicine" and receive its 'abundant rewards?'

FRY*:*

Medical practitioners are held in awe and deeply respected,
Therefore their pronouncements, as might be expected,
Are regarded as if divinely perfected.
Upon their authority there is erected
A belief that disease floats about until a victim is selected,
To be wretchedly and grievously affected.
Called contagion, the belief holds that we are infected,
By malevolent microbes that invade us quite unsuspected,
To wreak destruction upon us unless we are by vaccines protected.

Hence we hie to the medic we've elected,
To inoculate us with vaccine from a needle injected,
That we might henceforth by evil microbes be neglected.
Though of voodooistic origin contagion has been medically resurrected,
To ensnare a populace that invariable becomes dejected,
Because cures through medicine are never affected.
Until the sublime truth that similar organisms from nature defected,
Suffer similarly when life's laws are in like manner disrespected,
Disease will remain as long as bad life habits are uncorrected. [The Great AIDS Hoax, pp. 105]

ANDERSON: Wow! What a poem! ...My first wife died of cancer, over four years after 'they' gave her a 'death sentence.' She spoke to you by telephone and you warned her chemotherapy and/or radiation would likely bring on her earlier death. As it turned *out, you died before she did* — and you were not even sick! In 'retrospect,' what might you say to my late wife, Agnes, and to others who suffer the devastating trauma of a "cancer diagnosis?"

FRY: There are three areas in which we significantly short change ourselves: (1) Most of us fail to eat properly. We violate our physiological mandate or our biological adaptations with almost everything we eat. (2) Most of us fail to get enough vigorous activity to insure fitness. (3) Most of us fail to obtain enough sleep.

To say that most of us eat atrociously is to put it mildly. To put into ourselves all kinds of "junk" and expect to be healthfully nourished is tantamount to putting kerosene, vinegar or water into our auto fuel tanks and expect to get the high level of performance obtained from the best grades of gasoline. More than anything else, the quality of our lives is determined by the quality of our eating styles! [***Helping Hand: A Guide to Healthy Living***, 1990, p.3]

ANDERSON: Are you telling people they should trust a 'dead man's views' over our best trained, well-respected, highly paid medical professionals?

FRY: Why should you ever see a physician? They're called for only in case of serious accidents. Even so, their procedures are often harmful, even fatal. Drugging is a danger whether you're in sickness or health.

ANDERSON: I fancy myself a fruitarian; and, I feel in 'absolute' control of my health. But, I have been told, by other Natural Hygienists, that there could be dire consequences to maintaining a diet of mostly fruits. What do you say?

FRY: You're absolutely correct in eating fruits and their juices, in daily exercise, and presumably, getting adequate sleep, sunshine, fresh air and other of life's essentials.

Rest, like diet, is an essential of life. When partaking of food, it is wise to be in a well-rested condition so that your body can better devote itself to the appropriation and digestion of food.

A warm, loving, considerate, cheerful and happy mental disposition is a primary essential to best well being. General health, which includes fitness, predisposes to these positive qualities.

In pursuing fitness and health goals, a convinced and committed mind must precede the undertaking and prevail until ultimate death. [***HH: A Guide to Healthy Living***, pp. 120-122]

ANDERSON: What of migraine headaches, are they related to eating styles or diet?

FRY: Yes. Many migraine sufferers get their headaches due to food intolerance. Specifically thramines and other chemicals, which are found in chocolate, coffee, potatoes, peppers, egg plant and paprika. *Headaches result from a highly toxic bloodstream.* [***HH: A Guide to Healthy Living***, p. 102]

ANDERSON: Where can the public look — what can they read for themselves — to challenge or confirm your rather firm and narrow views?

FRY: Don't believe anything! Proceed only on verifiable facts. For instance, it stands to reason that a biologically correct diet is what you'd relish if returned to pristine nature from whence we came. Your senses direct you to the correct foods just as do [the senses of] other animals.

The truth is rather self-evident if we take natural perspectives rather than those of commercialized society. [***Helping Hand,*** pp. 119-120 #82]

ANDERSON: A lot of people know that Harvey and Marilyn Diamond, co-authors of the all-time best seller, ***Fit for Life,*** learned from you, and publicly acknowledged you as their teacher, their mentor, and as their most respected friend. Is there a 'common theme with other writers, thinkers, speakers, researchers, and scientists as well?

FRY: ***Knowledge is the greatest need of our benighted and purblind world. Knowledge of how to life; knowledge of the nature and purpose of disease; knowledge of the evils and futility of treatment; knowledge of the truth about life—this is the need of the whole world today.***

"My children are killed for lack of knowledge," says the god of the Hebrew scriptures. Millions die yearly because they lack true conceptions of life, of health, of disease, of cure. More people are killed every year by the causes of and the treatments for "disease" than by any other causes, only because their ignorance leads them to ignore causes and to rely upon "cures."

ANDERSON: Can you be more specific?

FRY: Education must supplant treatment; faith in the processes and forces of life must take the place of faith in "cures;" confidence in the normal things of life must displace confidence in abnormal things; trust in the laws of life must crowd out trust in vicarious atonements. Only thus can the ages-long frenzied search for "cures" be ended. Only thus can the terrible waste of time, money, energy and mental effort in the search for "cures" cease and all this time, money, energy, and effort be re-directed into profitable channels.

The frenzied search for "cures" must cease. ***Mankind must learn that the so-called disease, which they seek to cure, is, itself, the process of cure.*** All efforts to cure the cure are vicious and destructive. Unfortunately, the "healing" professions and the public still have the troglodyte's conception of disease. They still conceive of it as an attack upon the body by outside and unseen forces. The truth reaches them slowly. [***Program for Dynamic Health***, pp. 114-115]

ANDERSON: You lauded Prof. Peter Duesberg for his concurring views that "**HIV does not and, indeed, cannot cause" so-called AIDS** because "HIV appeared in only half of the full blown cases of AIDS." Yet, you express some disappointment in Professor Duesberg's quoting of Koch's postulates. Would you care to elaborate, please?

FRY: Dr. Duesberg is perhaps one of the foremost cancer and viral researchers in this country. His findings irrevocably say that the retrovirus called HIV not only does not cause AIDS but also *cannot* cause AIDS.

As an adjunct to his presentation, he printed Koch's postulates as altered by some unthinking medical mind (underscore added). Koch's postulates say: To establish a microorganism as a cause of disease:

1. It must be found in all cases of the disease.
2. It must be isolated from the host and grown in a pure culture.
3. It must reproduce the original disease when introduced into an unaffected organism, and...
4. It must be found present in the experimental host so infected. In short, the presence of the causative agency must always occasion the disease.

When I learned the postulates, the word *susceptible* was not in them. The medical system has interpolated this word into Koch's postulates as quoted by Dr. Duesberg. When anyone quotes the postulates with the word susceptible in them, they are not quoting Koch and, the use of the word susceptible destroys the proposition anyway!

The word susceptible was obviously interpolated to explain away the fact that experimental hosts rarely, in fact, almost never, come down with the disease the blamed agency was said to cause. ***The swabbing of noses with the nasal excrement of cold sufferers did not cause colds in the 1965 National Institute of Health cold experiments in Bethesda, Maryland.***

ANDERSON: What, exactly, is your point?

FRY: A cause, of course, is always a cause! If a blamed causative agency does not cause the disease it is supposed to cause when reintroduced into anyone, then it is not a cause.

The word susceptible means that the criterion which establishes susceptibility is the cause of the disease and not the microorganism or the agency blamed! That is just as clear and self-evident as the postulates themselves. The interpolation destroys the axioms.

I am surprised that someone of Dr. Duesberg's giant mental stature could overlook this. [***Hoax***, pp. 80-81]

ANDERSON: Dr. Fry, just what is disease? Is it anything more than dis-ease in the body politic?

FRY: If you live healthfully, you will appreciate only good health, for microbes will be symbiotic completely. The 'bad' bacteria and fungi are with us all the time, but in such a small number in those who live healthfully that, due to lack of nutriment, they do not generate significant amounts of poisons. Putrefactive bacteria are almost totally absent in the raw foodist living off our biologically correct diet of fruits with some vegetables, nuts and seeds.

ANDERSON: What 'causes' disease, whether real or imagined?

FRY: ***As causes of disease, neither bacteria nor fungi are basic to the process. Neither are so-called viruses.*** Even physicians unwittingly admit this.

Diseases are body initiated and conducted for the purpose of extraordinary detoxification and functional restoration. When regular channels of elimination cannot cope with the task for keeping the body clean, then a crisis called sickness is initiated to achieve cleansing and repair.

Physicians will tell you that bacteria, fungi and viruses are the causes — in those who are susceptible! That copout tells you that these agencies do not cause disease but those factors which dispose us to susceptibility do. Which is to say they do not cause disease at all. For what are called pathogenic bacteria, fungi and virii are always with us! If they caused disease, we would never be free of it. [***Hoax***, pp. 75-76]

ANDERSON: My new wife, Margie, is a Ph.D. in nursing, an R.N. and former Dean of Nursing at a famous American university in the South. She has joined forces with the **Organic Wellness Crusade (http://www.organicwell.com)** — my organization — to help spread 'the truth' to the world about "becoming sick, getting well." What advice would you give us, or what critical guidance would you suggest as the fundamental principle around which our efforts should focus?

FRY: The whole concept of medicine is downright myth. First, all detoxification and repair are inherently biological processes.

Nothing other than the organism has the intelligence, power and resources to heal. Hence, there can be no such thing as medicine. Thus no drug can or will help your ailment.

Drugs can only do specific harm, never good.

Keep this obvious truth in mind: you cannot be poisoned into health with drugs euphemistically called medicines.

ANDERSON: How does Natural Hygiene relate to allopathic medicine?

FRY: NATURAL HYGIENE is a way of life and has nothing in common with the so-called healing arts. Natural Hygiene holds that the organism is self-sufficient if supplied with its requirements, that is, fresh air, pure water, sunshine, exercise, wholesome foods, rest, sleep, security of life and its means, etc. Natural Hygiene rejects all drugs, medications and treatments, holding that they interfere with vital processes and are most often downright injurious. Natural Hygiene recognizes the plainly obvious in asserting that only the living organism can heal itself if injured or diseased. [***Program for Dynamic Health,*** copyright page, 1974]

ANDERSON: Forgive me if I seem to keep coming back to the same theme, but please bear with me. People in Africa and in other places, like The Bronx (NY), Dade County (FL), Appalachia (TN), Russia (EE) and many other places face daily starvation, homelessness, political neglect, religious abandonment, and public numbness. Why should these people even care about whether AIDS is a 'big lie' or not, or whether 'cancer' can be corrected by dietary modifications and body detoxification? Or, why should hungry, deceived, or disillusioned people care about any of this wellness stuff?

FRY: The primary reason that our statistics show greater longevity is because infant survival rates are now so high. A hundred years ago an infant was lucky to survive the birth and first year. However, those reaching one year of age were just as likely to reach 80 years of age as today.

Today's infants, though worse fed than a century ago, are not subjected to the filth, deadly drugs, and unhealthful practices of a century ago.

Despite establishment efforts to confuse, obfuscate and hamstring health seekers, a greater percentage are consciously embracing better practices than ever before in history. Today our enlightened people are eating more fruits and vegetables and less of harmful foods and than ever before.

ANDERSON: You seem to be suggesting Natural Hygiene—implementing wholistic lifestyles—is having a significant impact on a segment of the population. Am I correct?

FRY: This is not to praise a sizable segment of our society that is eating worse than ever before.

People are growing larger than ever before for the same reason our chickens; cattle and hogs are growing larger. Just as chickens, hogs and cattle are routinely fed hormones, antibiotics and other drugs that distress the organism, thus causing premature development, excess fat and giantism, so too do humans who are subjected to these or similar substances respond by unwholesome gigantism, premature development of sexual faculties and abnormal weight. [***Helping Hand***, pp. 110-111]

ANDERSON: Is good health, or healing, only for the rich, the 'educated,' the housed, the controlling segments of societies?

FRY: Healing—restoration of health, wholeness, integrity—is normal, a physiological or biological process. It results from the orderly operations of the ordinary and regular forces and processes of life, working with agents and substances that bear a normal relation to the living organism. Success of the body's efforts at self-healing depends absolutely upon removal of the cause of its ills. This is to say, the body cures itself when cause is removed. There is no cure outside of correction of cause.

ANDERSON: Then, how can ordinary citizens—of whatever country, state, county, city, neighborhood, or village—take charge of their own well-being?

FRY: The purpose of this volume is to awaken you to some easy-to-apply methods that will yield you sufficient rewards to spur you further along the course of learning our bodies' and minds' requirements. That this is easy is evident: Animals in nature without any special learning whatsoever instinctively observe their biological adaptations. In your case as, indeed with most others, the need is for deprogramming yourself of habits that sabotage your well being, and learning to do what you should have been doing all along.

Because it is such an easy and such a key change to make, this volume emphasizes food-combining principles. Harmonious digestion decrees that we so combine our foods that they are compatible in digestive chemistry. Failure to do this has built a billion-dollar antacid industry and made Tagament one of the best-selling drugs. It has been said that about 50% of the meals partaken in this country beget indigestion. [***HH***, pp.3-4]

ANDERSON: But, how will people in various countries know what to do, or what to eat?

FRY: The question implies some assumptions that are not necessarily so. China, with the world's greatest population, is actually fed on fruits, vegetables, tubers, grains, and roots with very little fish and meat in the diet. And they are decreasing their population.

Vegetarian populations are less warlike regardless of crowding, though the pressures of over-population have been attributed as a cause of war.

Long life does not lead to overcrowding. There are several countries in the world where the populace is appreciating greater longevity, yet has zero population growth.

Vegetarian populations are less, not more, disposed to wars. [***HH***, p.118#77]

ANDERSON: Most people in the world have been taught they cannot live, healthfully, without animal protein in the diets. What do you say to them?

FRY: Fish and meats, with their heavy complement of fats and proteins, are difficult to handle. This is why Eskimos usually die at age 40 to 50 years. Their kidneys and other organs just give out trying to cope.

Fish and meat are not essential items of diet anywhere in the world. [***HH***. P 118 #76]

ANDERSON: All my life I have lived, thought, and acted and believed as an 'optimist.' Now, after your untimely death, I am a bit cynical as I attempt to complete this volume we started out to write together (me, with your assistance and involvement). Is there any hope in continuing a <u>crusade</u> to help people see the simple but ***'absolute connection' between their lifestyle behaviors and their lifestyle 'diseases?'***

FRY: As you are undoubtedly aware many people are stubborn and cling to their erroneous concepts, their bad habits and injurious practices in the face of all reason. **Some even hold tenaciously to killing habits with the knowledge they are doing so! Life is not precious to them.** This attitude alone is life defeating.

This speaks not to spineless creatures so much as it speaks of a sick society, of humans in the aggregate who are

so perverted, so depraved and so degenerated that there is seemingly, no hope for them.

Yet I am not convinced the case for America is hopeless. **It is better to try in vain than not to try at all.** I am persuaded that the majority of Americans would wholeheartedly embrace the valid health practices of NATRUAL HYGIENE if they could be induced TO THINK, ever so little, FOR THEMSELVES! I feel that, if they could see the problem, THE TRUE STATE OF THINGS, and the simple solutions, they would awake from their lethargy and adopt the proper courses in life.

ANDERSON: Dr. Fry, the task is a momentous one...to say the least! It drains every personal resource, and frankly, I sometimes ask myself, 'What's the use?"

FRY: The problem is a gigantic one! I know that YOU will do what you can to help when you realize its seriousness. Every conscientious individual who sees the grievous wrongs in America is bound to devote some of his energies and resources to helping correct them.

*Americans must be made aware that ignorance in itself is not their obstacle but that they know so much—**so much that is not true!*** [***Program For Dynamic Health***, pp. 16-17]

ANDERSON: Let me ask you more directly: Why should anyone choose (a) discontinuing 'causative pleasures,' (b) detoxification, (c) therapeutic fasting, (d) rest; and, (e) 'attempting to' not poison themselves (with medications) into health, rather than just continuing to believe medical dogma that says: (1) innocent people become sick; (2) research, tests and drugging can cure dis-ease; (3) the masses are endangered because of the 'contagious nature of infectious diseases;' and (4) that surgery, chemotherapy, radiation, medications, and combinations of these are the treatments of choice for both non-degenerative and for degenerative disease conditions in 'developed societies?"

FRY: Good health in America is a downright myth! Contrary to what the medical profession, the press, radio and TV, in fact, our commercial masters would have us believe, (in

1974) health in America is in a woeful state. We realize less than half our true potential, and much of our shortened lives is plagued with life sapping economic insecurity, chronic disease, tormenting hopes and general suffering.

Lest you underestimate the gravity of the problem or the extent of suffering and ruinous practices in America consider these unpleasant facts ***[Note: the following statistics are quoted as of the year 1974; these data are multiplied in the year 2002!]:***

1. The U.S. Public Health Service recognizes a mere, 3,000,000 of our over 210,000,000 population as being healthy! This is about 1.5%!
2. 54% of all Americans die of heart disease! Over 50 million Americans suffer from severe heart disease. Autopsies of our most fit young men who died on the Korean battlefields show that 77% of them already had heart disease! Biologists state that a healthy heart should serve the human organism for at least 300 years!
3. About one billion visits are made to physicians annually in the U.S.A.!
4. About 4,500,000 people each year are poisoned so seriously by their physicians to require hospitalization! Tens of thousands die! The so-called side effects or adverse reactions of drugs are perfumed language for POISON EFFECTS! All drugs or "medicines" are inherently poisonous!
5. The U.S. ranks 89th among nations in death rate!
6. One out of every four Americans will have cancer! Cancer is the number one cause of death of our children! WHY? There are some countries where almost no cancer exists.
7. Arthritis and rheumatic complaints will effect 77% of our adult population!
8. About 40,000,000 Americans suffer allergies!
9. 60% of the population suffer defective vision!

10. Over 79,000,000 Americans are obese, far more than half of Americans are over-weight, yet nearly all Americans are malnourished in one way or another despite gross overeating!

11. 103,000,000 Americans (49%) suffer from AT LEAST ONE chronic disease or disability!

12. Over 30,000,000 Americans will spend some time in a hospital each year!

13. 50% of Americans suffer from digestive disorders.

14. An estimated 25,000,000 Americans suffer from high blood pressure.

15. Over 7,000,000 children are mentally retarded, disturbed or otherwise seriously handicapped.

16. 98.5% of our population has bad teeth! 31,000,000 have no teeth of their own! Filling, dental cavities, decayed and deformed teeth are so prevalent that they are considered normal! The average American child has six cavities by school age! Good teeth have the possibility to serve the human organism for several centuries with breakdown!

17. Over 20,000,000 Americans suffer from mental illness!

18. Life expectancy of a one-year-old is no more today than is was in 1900. Life expectancy is actually decreasing in the U.S.A.! Scientific studies indicate that a one-year-old can expect to live no longer than our ancestors did 10,000 years ago!

19. 58.6% of America's children cannot pass a physical fitness test!

20. Over 50,000,000 aspirins are taken daily in the U.S.A. This amounts to about 20,000,000 pounds of aspirin yearly! What a kind-size headache America suffers!

21. Nearly all Americans (almost 100%) suffer from digestive leukocytosis and a pathologically high heartbeat.

These conditions are largely the results of a pathogenic diet, drug habits and lack of healthful practices.

22. **Over 200,000,000 Americans are hooked on one or more drug habits!** (Emphasis this writer's). The drugs of most frequent use are caffeine, nicotine, alcohol, salt, aspirin, theine, theobromine and vinegar.

23. Nearly 100% of American women suffer debilitating leukorrhea and its consequent monthly hemorrhaging. Unfortunately this disease is regarded as normal in women of childbearing age.

24. Over 3,000,000,000 (that's three billion) sleeping pills are consumed annually. An estimated 13,000,000,000 barbiturate and amphetamine pills are ingested annually! Tranquilizers are a way of life!

25. Nearly 20,000,000 Americans submit to the surgeon's knife each year!

26. Murders, suicides, juvenile delinquency, narcotic addiction and other forms of crime are rife and increasing! A sick people make a sick nation.

ANDERSON: In all fairness, Dr. Fry, your statistics go back to 1974! What is the year 2002 picture expected to be like?

FRY: I could give you a seemingly endless resume of such statistics but why go on? The National Center for Health Statistics of the U.S. Public Health Service publishes volumes that reflect the widespread pathology of Americans.

Tell me, does this describe a healthy or a happy nation?

I hope that you're convinced that good health in America is a myth, that matters are in a terrible state and that something constructive MUST BE DONE! [***Program for Dynamic Health,*** pp. 19-21]

ANDERSON: Dr. Fry, my most respected and beloved mentor, your love and concern for others continue to show, even **from your 'final resting place.'** I thank you, on behalf of all of us. As this 'interview' draws to a close between **you, who died on September 6, 1996,** and me, who struggles still into **the next Millenium,** may I ask you for any final thoughts?

FRY: ...So ominous are the problems that beset America that I ask you to adopt a sane program of health practices as advocated herein. It is with a deep sense of purpose and commitment that I urge you to do what you can to help the Society (**American Natural Hygiene Society**) spread and perpetuate its program for bringing good health to America! There is much you can do, as you'll learn.

ANDERSON: As humankind transitions into Millennium 2000, what wellness orientation would best serve this and future generations?

FRY: ***The medical system is an outright failure! For some 2,500 years it has been trying to give man dispensation for his health transgressions without success.*** It has been trying to salvage him from disease through medication (drugs) while man continued to indulge the injurious practices that resulted in disease.

Today there is a veritable army of medical practitioners and a far larger corps of support personnel. They have an arsenal of drugs, potions, pills, medicines, vaccines, serums, antibiotics and "miracle" treatments. They constantly seek new and "better" remedies, for, in all this time, they have not succeeded in vanquishing A SINGLE DISEASE, though they take credit for conquering many!

Despite all the "miracle" drugs and "scientific" discoveries, they are faced with a growing army of the diseased. Hospitals are built in ever increasing proliferation. Physicians are being trained by the thousands. Nursing candidates are being assured of employment even before their training begins. ARE WE DESTINED TO BECOME A NATION OF SICK PEOPLE?

Why does the multitude of the suffering continue of grow? Why do their illnesses become ever more complicated? Why are such disabling diseases as cancer and arthritis on the upsurge? Why do more and more of our people die of cancer and heart disease?

IS THE DETERIORATING HEALTH OF AMERICANS A TESTIMONIAL TO THE VALIDITY OR THE INVALIDITY

OF THE MEDICAL SYSTEM? Will you think about that for a moment?

ANDERSON: I have thought about that question, Dr. Fry; and I tend to agree with you. But, what can challenge our 'great minds,' especially celebrities, powerful people, scholars, devout religious people, and families who feel victimized, especially when they hold charity events, walk-a-thorns, and even bake sales, believing they are helping by raisings funds for research, research to find cures?

FRY: For 2,500 years the highest powers of the human mind have been devoted to the invention or discovery of cures for the diseases of man. Many of the brightest minds have engaged in this search. Untold mountains of wealth have been poured into the effort to find cures.

For the past fifty years, "scientists" have devoted so much time, energy, talent and technical knowledge to this search that it makes all preceding efforts in this direction pale into insignificance. The whole field of nature has been ransacked to discover antidotes for the many diseases with which man suffers.

The chemist has analyzed every substance of nature, both organic and inorganic. He has created combinations as varied and numberless as the leaves of the forest. Not a mineral or a vegetable poison, however virulent, has escaped being tried or added to the truly frightful load of medicines to be used to cure man's diseases. The poisons of insects, of spiders, of snakes, as well as the excretions and pusses of animals have been added to the *materia medica*. Can any sane person believe these are the elements of health?

In the hope of discovering some panacea or some specific cures for the ills of man, ambitious men have added thousands of drugs, or poisons, to the armamentarium of physicians.

Fortunes of tremendous magnitude have been acquired by the compounders of elixirs and cordials. Specifics galore have been announced with much hullabaloo. They have been tried and then gone their way—to give rise to new drugs. The results of all this searching and experimenting have not been fruitful. The search is now more feverish than ever! Ever greater expenditures are made. Yet diseases have increased; their malignancy and fatality have become more fearful. Chronic diseases, in particular, have enormously increased in modern times.

ANDERSON: What you say is more disturbing than it is enlightening. This kind of information forces people to consider whether they have been lied to all their lives. How can people reconcile this dilemma? What practical data are available?

FRY: There are in this country more than 360,000 physicians (in 1974!); there are thousands upon thousands of hospitals, clinics, sanitoria; there are many giant chemical industries turning out drugs and vaccines; there are thousands of wholesale and retail drug companies, employing an army of pharmacists; there is a great army of nurses, technicians and others who depend on the drug trade for their livelihood. In addition to all these, there are the manufactures of bottles, pillboxes, cartons and plastics, and there are the newspapers, magazines, radio and television that derive millions out of advertising these pernicious products. The drug industry, directly and indirectly, accounts for incomes and profits that run into many billions of dollars a year in this country alone. Yet, we are poverty stricken when it comes to good health!

ANDERSON: Given these heavy, burdensome statistics, what hope can you offer society?

FRY: Pitted against the bleak picture of disease that afflicts humanity is the greatest health discovery of all time—NATURAL HYGIENE—a way of living based on natural principles that enables human beings to remain in good health throughout life, and to return to good health in all remediable cases, if they are ailing.

The great, simple and most sublime truth which NATURAL HYGIENE reveals is that, incorporated in every living organism itself is a great vital regenerative capacity as part and parcel of its very life, identical with, and inseparable from, its very existence, by which and through which the organism developed.

This vital power of the organism will, if not interfered with, always tend to keep the body in high functioning order—dynamic health! If an organism is diseased it will, permitted the opportunity, eliminate body wastes and accumulated morbid matters, repair and knit injuries, remove infirmities and heal its impairments.

ANDERSON: There are great minds out there—women and men—who do not agree with your assessment of Natural Hygiene, nor with the attributes you assign to it, as far as human health and well being are concerned. Are these people to be dismissed?

FRY: The foes of NATURAL HYGIENE (usually those who have a vested interest in disease!) have been unable to demolish a single one of its basic principles or to discredit a single one of its essential practices, but, on the contrary, have strengthened it by all their genuine discoveries!

Every advance of knowledge in biology and physiology has served to prove and confirm the scientific soundness of NATURAL HYGIENE and to remove the props from under the ancient practices of the medicine men.

ANDERSON: If you had to peer into the future, what would you say would be the ultimate outcome in this 'battle' to understand both the disease process and human well being?

FRY: Considering the vast importance of this body of truths and practices known as NATURAL HYGIENE and its role both restoring and preserving health it would seem that it would be more widely appreciated and cultivated. It is to this task that the Institute (Healthful Living Institute) applies itself and for which it asks your aid.

The facts of NATURAL HYGIENE are so incontrovertible, however, that eventually the most incredulous will be compelled to accept them. The strongest prejudice must ultimately give away before the crushing reality of HYGIENIC truth. [***Program for Dynamic Health***, pp. 22-26]

ANDERSON: Is the essential teaching the same, or is there something new or different from 1970 when you first embraced a Natural Hygiene lifestyle?

FRY: NATURAL HYGIENE teaches that all disease stems from NERVOUS EXHAUSTION, that is, the exhaustion of nerve energy of vital force. When the body's fund of nerve energy is overdrawn or under supplied the body can no longer properly conduct vital functions efficiently or effectively.

When functional power is lowered the body's ability to eliminate metabolic wastes and unwelcomed extraneous material is hampered or, to illustrate graphically, we might say these morbid matters become dammed up in the system. The body is no longer equal to the task of expulsion of normal or abnormal wastes.

When unwelcome substances remain in, the integrity of the body economy is threatened. The toxic load of unexpelled morbid wastes causes the body to resort to an emergency crisis to rid itself of a condition called toxemia or, very simply, toxic overload.

ANDERSON: Sounds like you are, again, describing 'the disease process!' If that is your intention, please—by all means—continue!

FRY: The emergency crisis to preserve bodily integrity through extraordinary cleansing efforts is exhibited as symptoms known as sickness, disease, illness, ailment, affliction or malady. In this abnormal state the small fund or remaining nerve energy is mustered to the task of body purification. Normal and emergency outlets for elimination of toxic matter are utilized. ***Their location and characteristics (Emphasis this writer's) label the form these crises of elimination take***. Their characteristics or symptoms are called variously colds, fevers, inflammations, catarrhs or a long list of maladies *ad nauseam* — some 20,000 names of maladies have been catalogued. To hygienists all these crises, regardless of symptoms and characteristics, excepting those involving organic degeneration, are pure and simple, ***toxemia***. The body is loaded with more poisonous matters than it can tolerate in its current state of vitality.

When the body has completed the task of purification; when the body has purged itself of its toxic overload; when the accumulation of noxious matters have been reduced to a level commensurate with functioning in the current state of vitality, the subject is said to be healed or is well again.

ANDERSON: How do hygienic practitioners fit in with the scheme?

FRY: Hygienists have formulated a system of health recognizing man's complete dependence upon nature and, therefore, the role of natural means in keeping us in a state of health and its agency in speedily restoring health if it is lost through our failure to live properly.

We can aid nature best in restoring health, in the event of its loss, by regeneration of our fund of nerve energy. This is best accomplished by not expending the small fund of nerve energy that remains but, instead, undertaking a physiological rest, A COMPLETE REST! This is known as a fast. **A fast is the complete abstinence from all food except the only three inorganic nutrients man is capable of utilizing, this is, pure water, fresh air and sunshine.**

NATURAL HYGIENE implores us to heed our natural requirements for well being and to indulge them prudently and wisely. This constitutes the science of correct living. [***Program for Dynamic Health***, pp. 30-32]

ANDERSON: Thank you, T. C., for all your guidance and inspiration; thank you for your boundless **research**; thank you for 'swimming upstream' against Establishment propagandizing, that many of us might have the opportunity to learn what is true.

On to a matter I consider personally important: *When I first learned of your death from a friend who had seen it flashed over the Internet, I immediately thought, "Foul play!"* Tell us, now, did your death result from 'accidental' or from orchestrated causes?

FRY: Did you know that you and the rest of your fellow citizens are victims of an ongoing fraudulent scheme on a scale so massive that it makes miniscule the collective criminal scene that we are aware of?

...In a nutshell, we are callously and mercilessly exploited and physically despoiled by a system that involves our subjection to and manipulation by the communications media (TV, radio, newspapers, magazines, etc.), the medical system, the banking system, the nation's production and distribution system and, ultimately, the master control system in this country, the Federal Reserve System, which is privately owned and controlled by the Rockefellers, Rothschilds, Kuhns, Loebs, Lehmans and a few other consorts. This article restricts itself to one facet of this cruel, dehumanizing and murderous fraud. It concerns ***a "myth"*** that was devised as a tool to keep us effectively servile and exploited.

Because this "myth" really was deliberately devised to ensnare us, it is more properly called a hoax. ***This hoax concerns a fictitious entity called a virus.***

A virus is an evil spirit! And that is about all that can be said of viruses to anyone who seriously tries to search them out. For what is called a virus is being blamed for more and more of our diseases. Now the move is on to attribute a viral cause to strep throat.

ANDERSON: *Dr. Fry, are you suggesting that your 'expose' of the so-called causal 'virus' could give rise to so clandestine a conspiracy as to order your 'neutralization' or murder?* I mean what is so revealing about a virus that it threatens the foundation of the hospital and pharmaceutical cartel?

FRY: A virus is said to be a minute bit of genetic material about a billionth the size of a cell (*per **Guyton's Textbook of Medical Physiology***). A virus is described as a genome surrounded by a capsid (covering) that is usually a double lipid/protein sheath. That seems to describe perfectly the genomes of the body's mitochondira too.

A genome (genetic material) is the pattern for directing the activities of a minute form of life known as a mitochondrion. The genome is endowed with the encoding that helps it create energy for itself and the cell, to create proteins of the kinds needed from amino acids, and yet other functions that maintain genetic integrity, like reproduction, for instance.

But imagine picking up books on microbiology, biology and virology and learning that virii (plural of virus) have these unlifelike characteristics:

1. They have no metabolism. They cannot process foods and have no energy formation. They're only a template or a pattern.
2. They have no faculties for action of any kind, no nervous system, and no sensing or decision-making faculties, much less movement and "invasion."
3. They cannot replicate themselves, depending wholly upon "obligate reproduction," that is, reproduction by an alien organism, something unheard of in all biology.

They are merely inert organic material without any life qualities whatsoever. They are never seen to act, and photographs purporting to show them acting are outright frauds, revealing no action whatsoever from the virus. What is usually shown is an ordinary process of phagocytosis (process of cellular ingestion) which occurs countless trillions of times daily in the body, perhaps more than a quadrillion times!

ANDERSON: I am not sure I am getting your meaning!

FRY: Have you ever heard of one organism actually reproducing another? Not another organism at that! A genome is not an organism, micro or macro. It is to a mitochondrion what a head is to the human body—a control mechanism. As this is contrary to all that we learn in biological science, it smacks of voodooism!

The medical (drug) establishment has taken a bit of mitochondrial debris and imbued it with the qualities of an evil spirit. They badly need a scapegoat for out ills. The success of that ploy is paramount for the merchandising of

their drug wares. The fact that acute diseases are body originated and conducted for the limited purposes of cleansing and repairing itself doesn't escape them, but that truth is bad for business. Healthy people are bad for business. ***And those who alert others to the sham are bad for business.***

ANDERSON: So, that's it: "...Those who alert others to the sham are bad for business" and are, therefore, expendable at the whim of others...?

FRY: ***But I want to assure you of one thing: You don't have to believe this! [HH***, pp. 1-2]

ANDERSON: With that, sir, I thank you from the bottom of my heart, and **I pray that eternal peace and inspiration will be always associated with your name and legacy!**

Author's Reminder:

This Anderson/Fry Interview was concluded on September 30, 1999 in the village of Igueben, Edo State, Nigeria (West Africa), some thirteen days after it began. The 'method of this interview' involved a student remembering his teacher: his teacher's context and his occasional inconsistencies; and it involved a re-reading of the teacher's published books, papers, newsletters, and other writings, in addition to reviewing some of Dr. Fry's contributions to other volumes, including this one. No 'hearsay' information was used (from interviews with persons who knew him well; and, perhaps, no one knew him better than Harvey Diamond, co-author of the all time wellness bestseller, ***Fit for Life***).

Questions were then posed with response spaces reserved. Appropriate responses were identified and inserted to fit the questions asked. None of T.C. Fry's words, syntax, or statements was altered to fit the questions asked. None of T.C. Fry's words, syntax, or statements was altered in any way. To the best of my ability, questions were posed that protected and supported the 'original' contexts from which quoted statements were pulled. If any juxtaposition is uncharacteristic, only this writer is to blame.

The motivation for this 'mock interview' was to permit this writer (Dr. Fry's student) to isolate essential, if not critical, viewpoints that epitomize the character and central mission of the man who called himself, simply, "Mr. Fry."

As a final gesture of love and respect, this writer dedicates the following poetic expression to the family, friends and admirers of the late T.C. Fry, D.Sc., Natural Hygienist, and personal guru.

GOODBYE, MR. FRY

Goodbye, Mr. Fry…goodbye!
Why do I cry…when I think of how you died?
Why does it pain, to read more truth…about my hero?
Why did T. C. die so young?

That question belongs to others;
I know Jesus lived only to age 33;
JFK to age 42; MLK to age 39;
And Robert was not far behind!

I know that Malcolm X was, too,
"Very young," and Medgar was not old.
T. C. was 69 when he died.
What an 'old man' was he!

I miss him—as I did earlier on—
As a friend and a human person:
Fiery and full of energy (a 'visionary,'
Always pushing forth on some personal mission)!

"Not terribly realistic about business (ventures),"
but optimistic, to be sure.
Perhaps, even misguided by his own creative juices—
Or, by the influencing juices of others.

I knew T. C. Fry, the fruitarian, the Natural Hygienist,
Who would go any distance, anytime, to whisper
Into a Seeker's ear, about Dr. Herbert M. Shelton and
Natural Hygiene, the science of healthful living!

He, like Jesus, perhaps was a "misfit"—
Out of sorts with many of his contemporaries.
Thank God for that—for them both!
Yet, I tear up now and again.

I think I want to…until I try stopping.
Then, I smile of his memory; and he smiles back.
I miss him, you know; I loved him so….
He delivered, gave me 'freedom' (put into my hands manageable options).

I was empowered by his admonitions;
He answered most of my important questions.
He made me a part of himself; he saw good in me.
He was bigger, even bigger than himself.

People showed me "who" he was;
But I had little to do with 'that' person.
And so, I came to be ever so aware:
There were at least two "T. C. Frys!"

Now, there are none, except on paper and in memory.
Yet, there remains the man I knew…
The man I am still coming to know.
Still, he speaks to me; and I tend to hear more than he says.

Many "saw" his or her own 'version' of this man.
He was all 'those people,' but none of them, really….
He once told me I was 'needed' because I knew "how to keep it simple."
At this very moment, I am moved to be so advised.

T. C. has been martyred—by the circumstances of his life.
He championed Natural Hygiene, to the end—

Fighting as best he could, enervation and well-meaning friends.
Both can get you killed—as they too often do!

Accepted or not, Terry died slowly;
It took 69 years, years, years.
That was a long time, a long lifetime!
Now, I must say, again, 'Goodbye, Mr. Fry.'

Chapter Thirteen

What 'Disease' Really Is: Final Perspective

'Disease is **action;** it is on-going activity. It is symptom-producing; it is on a mission (as preordained as human existence itself!). *Disease is one Divine 'instrument' employed to 'recycle' human tissue.* Disease is the 'outcome' of years of poorly managed toxicity.

The human organism self-manages a fair and reasonable amount of internal poisoning; it eliminates what it must; and, *it stores the balance.* This is why so many "disease conditions" fail to make 'an appearance' until later in life. However, in the current age, "later in life" takes on a crude and frightening presence when we consider that the most dreaded disease of all—cancer—is the number one killer of our children (who, obviously, have not attained many years of age!). Why is this so, you ask? Allow your eyes to freely flow around the supermarket check-out stand, and observe what items are there to attract children. Take the family on a ride, or walk down "Main Street" and observe what "eating establishments" are cooking up for your children! Remember how 'special days' for children are celebrated; now, consider how deadly is all that sugar: how nutrient-deplete is all that starch, dairy, salt, oil, fat, seasoning, not to mention the fish, chicken, beef and pork!

Children die of cancer (internal poisoning) because "Wall Street" (advertising) and "parents" (all conspiring adults!) help to kill them! In a sense, you could say, "We <u>love</u> our children to death!"

It would be different if adults were equally vigilant about "detoxifying" children's internals. But, we learn too late, most never learning enough to serve themselves in a timely manner. Only a new, don't-give-a-damn-about-what's-easy-but- about-what's-healthy breed of parents will spare children the 'modern curse of death by cancer (called by many and sundry names!).

In developing countries, the picture changes to economic deprivation, poverty, malnutrition (now passed off as "AIDS"), starvation, and discrimination that 'excludes' having the rest of the world know the truth. Inoculations which years later are called "A.I.D.S." effectively insulate human compassion from for what in effect, is nothing short of "materialism, greed and the love of money," says my daughter, Brenda. And, I agree. *Peoples with melanin* "suspect" they are "under attack" but often cannot figure out quite how (though they often feel they know 'why.').

The irony is that people of the Caucasian (***non-melanin***) race are 'programmed' for obsolescence, because the vast world-wide health care industry derives the vast majority of its funding from other Caucasians. It's like the story told in bars about the couple making love on the railroad tracks, with a train coming. "So are we!" They shout. Who dares to stop this flow?

'Slavery' continues in America—transferred to the Caucasian community: drugs /drug addition (usage) is a white, middle class phenomenon. Despite the *"urban-poor-ghetto-people" with melanin* broadcasting that goes on, the reality is that white, middle class women consume the lion share of drugs bought and paid for in America (some 70%!). That white women are so addicted is no accident; *but it is 'political!'*

The obsolescence of white people is further orchestrated in dietary patterns (principally in meat and dairy consumption [just look at yogert, for example!] that lead to and insure impotence in white males and sterility in white females; the net result is a negative birth rate (more Caucasians dying than are being born). An average math student can 'predict' when the white race will literally 'expire,' if the present trend is not reversed.

The Nature of Disease

When there is the obvious presence of disease in the human organism, we are observing the evidence of neglect. What we are seeing are the 'symptoms' (the stuff upon which medical examinations, medications and procedures are built!) of toxic overload. How many ways can this simple fact be stated?

Now enter (again!) vision of The Grand Reaper (Mother Nature, God, The Creator) "ushering in" the effect of cause, the 'natural consequence' of too much poison in the system. Remember our earlier discussion about bacteria and germs? How the role of germs was to return organic matter back to Nature? Yes, you got it! Eschatologically speaking (a theological term meaning loosely "at the end of human/spiritual existence") what we know as "disease" (by all its various names) is nothing more or nothing less than "an aging or universal action for facilitating the transition of organic matter from its present stage to its ultimate stage [as far as we generally pursue the matter])."

The Purpose of Disease

The late, great, T.C. Fry said that what we call disease is "self-initiated, reparative activity" by the organism, in an effort to restore well being. Dr. Shelton, John H. Tilden, MD, Dr. Alec Burton, Harvey Diamond, and many others concur, adding that "only the body has the innate intelligence to heal itself."

Of course, I believe as my gurus believe and wrote; but, inspired by their insight I "see" that **the body will not heal itself** unless the individual person (or a human intercessor) successfully manages (to sufficiently reduce) the level of toxicity stored in the body and/or the mind. Failing to so manage the amount of poison within, the body (disease) knows but one course of action: to return **this** organic matter back to Mother Nature (almost always, prematurely)!

We call it 'death' but that is our myopic view. This taught-perspective fails to comprehend the 'Celestial' reality—the

Cosmic Truth: organic substance does not "die." It transforms to another state and is, in fact, eternal. Living souls (our organic essences) do not die, "personalities" do. The electrical elements formerly known as "John Doe" just transition or transform to universal elements, rejoining Existence as it is fundamentally maintained in the Universal Scheme of Creation. What this says, also, is that disease is as much a part of living as it is of dying; and, in either eventuality, it is "neutral" or 'unbiased.'

"Just say no to drugs" is the "honey that catches the flies!" The drug culture in poor communities is a well-publicized tragedy, a major vehicle for imprisoning young persons of color. Yet, **the real tragedy in America is the murder of white women, the owners of American wealth** (even though men control this wealth)! White women purchase some 70% of the Three Trillion Dollars in drug revenue; and white women are the most terrorized, then killed (murdered) by medical testing, prescribing and treating. Medical procedures mask cardiovascular effects of 'tolerated' lifestyles and "cancer treatments," the number one and number two killers of women in Western society. But, we are 'encouraged' to believe it is men who die more frequently from "heart disease."

White male domination determines who lives and who dies; and there is no effective challenge to this paradigm—not yet anyway! This too might seem ironic but white women need men of color—for the survival of them both. Children would have ***melanin*** (protection from 'ozone layer poisoning') and they would have real caring. Single men would be spared unjust jailing and premature death. The prison system, while cruel and unjust, preserves lives that might not otherwise survive urban dynamics!

There is hope ahead, because Good shall emerge and "Truth, trampled to the ground, shall rise again!" said The Rev. Dr. Martin Luther King, Jr. Disease, as a sociological phenomenon, is a living challenge for society. Disease in the body is called 'poverty' in neighborhoods. **The purpose of either is**

destruction of the current, ordinary form of living—to, in fact, prematurely terminate existence.

Cycle of Life

By analogy, we could say our "life cycle" is like the face of a clock: life begins at 6, when we are born and ends at 6, when we "die" (transition, also referred to as "making our final transition"). Our individual **time line** moves left of 6, and the closer we are to the 6, the more vulnerable is our survival.

As we progress toward 9, then 12, one-quarter to one-half of our lives has been developing disease, or has been building internal toxicity—has been collecting garbage, both physical and mental. Either one and/or the other has but one pre-ordained mission: to hasten the final transition of this organic 'stuff' we call Henry L. N. Anderson, or Jacqueline Kennedy Onassis, or yourself.

Nor is there any 'judgment' made about this construct. It is because it IS; and it is quite consistent with the Universal Law of 'Effects of Cause.' Disease in organic matter (such as ourselves) can be likened unto rust which, if not well managed hastens metal's return to universal elements. In a sense, both rust in metal and disease in humans serve a similar function: they hasten the (most often premature) return or transition back to natural elements. Without disease, life goes merrily on for 150 years or more.

Natural Law governs all of Creation—here on earth and conceivably in the vast Universe as well. Part of this governing is managing the time line to the final transition of any element—human notwithstanding. Evidence of this fact is all around us. Sparrows and pigeons police city streets. Roaches and rats clear away exposed foodstuffs. Vultures keep dead carcasses 'transitioning.' Sharks dispose of dying and dead marine life; worms recycle a variety of organic fare; and an entire network of predators hasten the 'final transitions' of the young, the weak, the old, the dying, and the dead.

So, we humans can expect our time lines to be directly correlated to how well or how poorly we manage the development of poison build-up (disease) in our lives. It is this act of on-going management that determines how soon or how late we "deep six" (make our final transition), under normal circumstances (traumatic death not included).

As a co-existing consequence, the quality of one's life also hinges upon the quality of the management of the developing disease reality in our lives. **And while it might appear that God blessed us with a healthy body, or 'cursed' us with an unhealthy one, the truth is neither: human behavior begets relative wellness—in a former generation, in this generation, or in the next generation!**

Toxins retained by parents (more often the father!) limit the state of wellness parents deliver to children. If children are able to manage the 'handicaps,' their own offspring can receive a better 'heritage.' But, God did not do it! God is 'neutral' to our exercise of "free will" (even when decisions are made for the unborn child!).

The point of this line of discussion is simply this: there is no "cure" for disease, except successfully managing the level of internal poisoning. We in wholistic wellness refer to this as "prevention." Speaking of cancer in 1986 the ***New England Journal of Medicine,*** reported that after some thirty years of cancer research, medical scientists "are losing the war against cancer." This was sixteen years ago! Even then, the report was daring enough to assert that "the most promising areas are in *cancer prevention* rather than treatment."

One has to wonder if all medical research (spending in the name of "medical cures") is misguided at best, and fraudulent at worst! **What "cures" disease is effectively managing its development, nothing else!** Learning is an integral part of management. We learned to purify drinking water and cholera was effectively eliminated. It was not "cured." Given a polluted drinking water scenario and, presto! Cholera is alive and well—again!

Cancer, for example, like AIDS (the effects of consuming medicines and drugs!) will never have a "cure." Unless people change their lifestyle activities (how they believe and act) **cancer—or AIDS—will continue to do its job: hasten the time line of our "final transition."**

Human beings might be less passionate about this construct. And, perhaps, we would be were it not for the fact that "programmed ignorance" of this fact is the 'corner stone' of a multi-trillion-dollar-a-year industry. We call it the healthcare industry!

In the next chapter, I will offer practical suggestions. Readers of this type of volume generally get worked up, and often make tentative commitments to "change my lifestyle." Often, such change is stymied by insufficient information, lack of clarity, or honest confusion. We will attempt to clear up some of that, and provide guidelines you can live with, or at least understand. The idea is for you to be able—should you elect — to make intelligent decisions, for yourself, about yourself, and to yourself.

The frenzied search for "cures" must cease. Mankind must learn that the so-called disease, which they seek to cure, is, itself, the process of cure. All efforts to cure the cure are vicious and destructive. Unfortunately, the "healing" professions and the public still have the troglodyte's conception of disease. They still conceive of it as an attack upon the body by outside and unseen forces. The truth reaches them slowly. [Program for Dynamic Health, p. 115]

— T.C. Fry (1974)

Chapter Fourteen

Women and Weight

African women tend to "carry weight" in their hips. A world traveler will tell you that Indian women carry weight in their stomachs. So do African American women. Fact of the matter is both women and men "carry weight in their hips and stomachs." The reason this is so is that the body, in its own infinite wisdom, stores excess "fat" (more food than the body needs!). The best places for such storage are away from the vital organs. Thus, the hips, thighs, upper arms, stomach, legs, neck, and some of the back are the locations.

The interesting thing about such storage, however, is that one has to "pay rent" to maintain the cache! This "rent" is represented by (a) continuing to crave and continual storage of excessive fat (otherwise, the amount stored would reduce!); (b) the expenditure of vast amounts of nerve energy, just supporting the extra weight, and guarding the 'stuff' so as to limit its negative influence on surrounding body tissue (this stored fat captures poisons moving through the body and holds them in bondage; therefore, the longer "extra weight" is maintained the more toxic it becomes.); (c) over the course of time, the body and/or the mind are impacted by this "stored garbage" (commonly, we refer to these effects as diabetes, cardiovascular disease, nervous breakdown, 'chronic fatigue syndrome, blindness, stroke, arthritis, and the myriad of commonly known disease disorders).

The body is very reliable; it is nearly perfectly consistent. It uses what it needs, eliminates what it must, and stores the balance. And from this storage, over 90% of human disease develops. This is why it is as debilitating to "not forgive" as it is to smoke cigarettes! Harboring jealousy and envy are no less deadly than consuming large amounts of simple sugars (white sugar, honey, bread, bleached rice, flour pasta, candy, and alcohol). Hating—whether it is something, someone, or yourself—is as harmful as consuming drugs!

It has been said that some 85% of the work force is unhappy with their positions, assignments, supervision or other aspects of the work environment. Unhappiness and dissatisfaction are no friendlier than the "wrong drugs" prescribed by physicians ("iatrogenics" ["at the hands of doctors"] kills an estimated 325,000 people yearly in the U.S.A., mostly from patients being given 'the wrong drugs.').

Extra weight, then, is more than obvious fat, vibrating from one's hips or thighs. It is all the stuff referred to above, and more. To the limited extent that what "keeps the weight on" can be attributed to the consumption of food, this is easy to fix! Just commit to eating half as much (of whatever you daily consume). The Law of Effects of Cause is operational. You will begin to lose weight immediately. You have to; it takes an 'equal' amount of water coming into the flowing fountain to match that which flows out to keep the level of the water at the same point.

"Dieting" as an isolated action will not work for healthy 'weight control' because it is done out of context. Without a fundamental change in behavior—lifestyle, if you will—similar 'causes' will generate the same old 'effects.'

We said earlier that if you have a concern for your cholesterol level all you have to do is cut back and/or eliminate animal products from your diet. How complicated is that, since the only source of "bad" cholesterol is the fat from animal tissue?

Much of the problem in unsightly and uncontrollable weight gain (unhealthy at best and deadly at worst) is that people do not seem to understand the factors that contribute to the situation. If you look at people eating, you observe how little they chew their food. You see how quickly they drink liquids (some simply "washing down" barely chewed food, time and time again!). Next, you might observe the amount of food (on the first plate served, then on the second plate, and often on the third and subsequent servings!). Finally, you might notice the abundance of starches (bread, rice, pasta, gravy, salad dressings, potatoes, yams, and eventually desserts), very little green, leafy vegetables and no fresh fruits (always should be eaten before other foods!).

Food is usually cooked, most often fried, and is showered with condiments (salt, pepper, spices, hot sauce, vinegar, butter, oil, sugar compounds). **All of these things add up to the development of disease within the organism.** But, from a strictly weight perspective, perhaps the most noteworthy factor is **amount**. People who have a weight problem consume too much solid food and too much liquid. They forget that bodies of water are larger than bodies of land. The human body stores the excess—of solid and/or of liquid! Ever wonder why the first weight lost is water weight? The 'last weight lost' is also water. So subtle—and important—is this issue that we will devote an entire chapter to the "water-weight issue."

We know well the expression: "You can't have your cake and eat it, too!" We don't believe it. If we did, we would see that the opposite is also true: You cannot lose weight by adding more than you subtract! By eating and drinking less—even if you fail to do the exercising, get the fresh air, feel the positive vibes, reach the level of forgiveness you need to reach—you will, nonetheless, drop some weight. Everybody is just kidding himself or herself if you think women have more problems with extra weight than do men!

The amount of food consumed by 'the average American' in one day could easily be spread over two or three days; and, the person would improve his or her well being immensely. There is a lot of truth in the statement that "Americans are eating themselves into early graves!" Men, take notice: why do you suppose there are so many widows in this country? Who prepares the meals in American homes? Who tries to "please my spouse" by consuming far more than is required by the body? Who gets sick first, and dies earlier? Do wives "kill their husbands in their kitchens?" Let this be food for thought; and, know that either spouse or other family member eating in a 'competitive spirit' hastens the path to sickness, disease and premature death. It is the Law of the Universe. Husbands who do the "cooking" appear to generally outlive and be in a better state of health than their non-food-preparing wives.

Detoxifying the Body

When all is said and done; when spending on medical research becomes 'vulgar;' when the dying public becomes "damned tired of dying;" when intelligent people discover that they **are born to be healthy**, and no longer need rely upon 'professional liars,' only then will the truth become crystal clear: **stored physical and mental 'garbage' breeds what we know well as diseases.**

Once understood and accepted for the self-evidence of its truth, individuals who make 'detoxification' a part of their on-going daily consciousness will seldom, if ever, experience either sickness or disease conditions. In this way, they will let their lights shine, "so that others, seeing, may take heart."

Opinions held—for years and with passion—are difficult to modify. Passion has a way of crowding out reason; and behaviors that extol a high price (our wellness) are accommodated because of familiarity and comfort. We literally 'kill' ourselves doing what is perceived to be 'cool' or 'traditional.'

It requires almost a 'moment of weakness' or extreme curiosity that one dislodges his or her comfort zone (old habits) to ponder: "How does my body detoxify itself?" And, having asked the question, the best received 'answers' are frequently those that come in the form of fads or popular opinions. It has been proven time and again that people tend to prefer that which "tastes good" over what **is** good. Our children are taught early to prefer sweet candy over sweet strawberries!

Herein lies the problem that besets us all: our earliest years of life on earth taught us reliance upon "taste" (enhanced, usually, by white sugar!) rather than upon goodness (organically grown, uncooked fruits, vegetables, nuts, and seeds). Since grains and legumes often need processing and/or cooking, they constitute a secondary food supply.

Other than distilled or purified drinking water, the unprocessed juices of organic fruits and vegetables, just about everything else we might drink contributes to the 'garbage' collected inside the body, and therefore to the onset of disease in the body. All soft drinks—whether "diet" or regular—are lethal, especially to the delicate tissue of a child's body! Yet, observe how adults nearly "force feed" sodas to children (an act that should be as "illegal" as drinking alcohol before the age of 21)! ***Is it any wonder that cancer is the number killer of children in the United States of America?***

So, the obvious answer to "How do I detoxify my body?" is that you should stop polluting it! Once you stop adding poisons to your body (and are able to do the same for 'mental garbage'), you can move to the next step: reduce the level of toxicity harbored by your body (and mind).

Of all the products on the market that promise detoxifying assistance, there is only one that this writer endorses. It is called H.A.R.A., an acronym for **Hurdle Antechachexy Regenerative Agent.** It is organically grown and sold without any additives, including preservatives and colorings. It has no taste enhancement and contains distilled or carbon-filtered water. It's "magic" is its prescription: how it is used! The results speak for themselves, as many individuals will testify.

H.A.R.A. (also a Japanese word meaning "life force") is marketed by the Organic Wellness Crusade (http://www.organicwellness.com). Aside from organically grown FVNS (fruits, vegetables, nuts and seeds), this is the only product of any description that is endorsed by this writer, other than distilled drinking water. One reason is the belief that stuff essential for the body should come from our food supply; the other reason is that ***H.A.R.A.* is organically grown in California by this writer**! It qualifies as an aid to well being because it "interferes least with the body's normal self-cleaning activities."

True detoxifying begins with 'prevention' and moves to the near complete elimination of stuff stored too long within the internal systems of the body. Just as it takes more than ten (10) years for "cancer" to manifest in the adult body, it might take as long to cleanse the body of old garbage. Yet, this cleansing remains one's best chance for avoiding catastrophic illness or disease conditions, earlier or later in life.

Put simply, stop poisoning yourself! **Know and believe**: soft drinks are not a healthy food substitute ("diet sodas" are a 'mirage,' giving an illusion of being 'better than regular sodas'); sweetened and cooked foods are disease-causing; animal fats (flesh foods) are the only source of harmful cholesterol; coffee and tea contain stuff that contributes to heart disease; dairy products can hardly be proven as a good food for human consumption; alcohol and drugs (spices and condiments) are forms of sugar and toxins. Other than putrefying animal protein, breads, desserts, and other "simple sugars" are the leading contributors to diabetes and associated illnesses and premature deaths!

Yet, Harvey Diamond (***Fit for Life***) makes a considerable argument for modestly indulging not only some dairy, but some animal flesh as well in his book, ***You Can Prevent Breast Cancer!*** This writer believes Harvey and Marilyn Diamond leaned toward uncertainty in their former book and that Harvey Diamond leans toward popularity in his recent book. Most recently, however, I believe he sharpens the line (at least privately).

People become "confused" because those who know and advise 'market' in creating confusion. "People do not want to know the bare truth!" they exclaim. Tell a person a truth that he does not want to hear and he will castigate you; tell him an untruth that he wants to hear and he revels you! So, the beat goes on....

Because we do not, and indeed cannot control our external environments, the 'genius' of a wellness lifestyle is that it does control whatever it can! People get sick who do not know why they are getting sick periodically. People who know do not get sick! People become diseased and often die prematurely because they do not understand what is happening to them. People who understand the 'process' take decisive steps, even if they begin them late in their lives!

Have you had contact with a person whose breath was very offensive, and reminded you of "a garbage dump?" Have you experienced the smell of body gas that caused you to immediately think of "something dying?" Or have you entered a lavatory and declared: "God, it smells like somebody died in here!" There is some truth in each scenario; internal garbage is evidence of "decay and death." Whether air passes over this decaying matter out of one's mouth or one's anal passage, it is the same evidence! Foul smelling body gas is Nature's way of warning the individual that his or her organism is in trouble; and, activities that enhance body cleansing should be commenced or increased. At the least, it is "no joke" to smell like something dead!

Such smells are warnings; they do not equate to the dynamics that take place within the cells themselves. Garbage stored in the body is stored all over the body, throughout the lymphatic system; it is contained in body fat; it is intermingling with cell structures themselves. This garbage is poison, toxicity. John H. Tilden, M.D., wrote a book entitled, ***Crisis of Toxemia,*** and that was Dr. Tilden's definition of "disease!"

While detoxifying the body implies "internal cleansing," it is not so simple a task as "flushing a toilet!" Colon cleansing notwithstanding, no single action or maneuver can 'cleanse' the human organism. Can one act of forgiveness clear up all the mental garbage stored over years? Can one long, organic or hygienic fasting experience eliminate all the 'stuff' built-up over several years? Is ethnic hatred removed by one act of inter-ethnic marriage?

Detoxifying is as much a way of living, an entire lifestyle pattern, as consumption is the source of all disease conditions. Even poisons in the atmosphere and in our environments—that we cannot control—must be *consumed* by our bodies for us to experience any negative effects. As trite as it may sound any detoxifying action must begin with "stopping" the daily acts of poisoning ourselves that we engage. Once we significantly stop or cut back on consuming toxins, or stuff that becomes toxic once consumed, we "reduce our risk of developing disease symptoms."

Two other factors are critically important in the detoxifying strategy of one who is determined to know the truth: (1) The human body must be constantly well exercised; the mind must be 're-programmed to the positive.' (2) What is consumed (physically and mentally) must enhance, not interfere with the organism's ability to utilize and to eliminate. What is not utilized is stored; what is stored is, obviously, not eliminated. And out of this "retained toxicity" comes conditions and symptoms matching every named "disease" in the ***Merck Manual***, the official reference that tells doctors what symptoms should be treated with which drugs!

'Treating' Any Known "Disease"

Supported by the writings of Dr. Herbert M. Shelton and John H. Tilden, MD, primarily, this volume advances the notion that "all diseases are the same disease," and "what remedies one disease, remedies all diseases!" Followed to its logical conclusion, no one needs fear becoming sick or "coming down with any degenerative or chronic disease." Of course, **prevention** is the key. If you can prevent poisoning yourself, and control the retained poison you could not prevent, surely there will be little or no place in your life for the onset of disease.

Nor is it hard or impossible to do. Perhaps the most critical ingredient is personal *commitment*. To become committed, one must first become enlightened. Questions must be asked, and answers must "make common sense." Simple tests must be made; and reasonable 'proof' must be visible. Actions must be replicated and the results must be consistent. It is out of this 'verifying process' that one comes to rely upon what the senses confirm is true.

Does a person continue to eat ice cream when it causes immediate and violent cramps in the stomach? Does one insist on eating chocolates at the expense of ugly pimples on the face and other body parts? Do people drink alcohol, become drunk, end up in a jail or a hospital only to sober up and restart the process? Do drug users steal and lie over and over again to acquire their drugs? "Yes" answers all of the above questions, but only until these individuals "decide" (become committed to the proposition) that **enough is enough**!

Now you know why my ***Helping Hand: 8-Diet Programs*** book has the expanded title: ***For People Who Care About Wellness*** (Publius Publishers, 1986). It matters not what the ailment or by what fancy name the set of symptoms might be called, **the cause is the same and the remedy is the same**. All diseases have their genesis in internal body filth, toxic substances warehousing within the body politic. Getting rid of this 'stuff' (as quickly as practical) is second only to preventing the build up in the first instance!

If this 'effects of cause' picture is not clearly seen, someone has 'blinders' on. If 'absolute proof' is required, do your own investigation. Ask older people to describe their earlier lifestyles. Just listen to what you hear. Visit patients at your local hospitals; sit down and chat with them. While you provide them comfort, they will fill you with information. You will begin to see a pattern, the inevitable consequences of consumption, storage, and the development of disease symptoms.

Finally, take out your notebook and record the daily eating and drinking habits of children. See how many days pass before they show signs of "having a cold." Pay special attention to how little rest they get; to how little balanced exercise they engage. Count the number of sugar-laden "foods" they consume throughout the day. Notice their general disdain for live foods: fruits, vegetables, nuts, seeds (raw, not roasted, unsalted). Take special note of how infrequently children eat anything green (a live food, as in uncooked vegetables!). See how much tension they endure; how much noise; and, if you can, anticipate their anxieties (the fallout of various forms of violence in their lives!). Measure the amount of sugar/caffeine liquids (soft drinks) they consume. Again, this writer asks: Is it any wonder more children die of cancer than from any other cause of death in the United States of America?

Chapter Fifteen

Weight Control: The Salt Connection

When the question of weight arises, invariably the conversation goes to diet. With any suggestion of weight control—whether weight reduction or weight gain—the immediate focus is generally, "What diet are you on?" or "What diet regimen do you recommend?"

In reflecting upon the weight control issue over the years (and observing how many of my first cousins are obese—women and men!), I have come to realize that there is almost "an invisible villain" co-responsible for the "crime" of overweight; but, heretofore, this villain has not been singled out, accused, and indicted for complicity in the "criminal offense" of causing the body to carry more than normally required body weight.

But, let us identify the accused. First, let us look at the most frequently accused elements in the diet: animal protein, animal fat, sugars, calories (carbohydrates, starches, etc.), and a variety of condiments. The picture is not yet complete. A principal player is ***water***! While we have all heard about "water weight," it usually appears in the professional trainer's or other professional's statement that "the first weight lost is water weight."

We have heard little about water weight as, perhaps, the first weight gained. One reason for this oversight might be that so little information is published that focuses on the role that the overall ***consumption and retention*** of water plays in weight gain.

A subtle, but critically important new factor enters the picture, and our minds expand slightly. Another "slight of hand" nearly missed being 'detected.' More will be said.

Let us look more closely at the water connection to overweight. When we look at seriously obese individuals—those weighing 500lbs, 700lbs, even 1000lbs—we wonder to ourselves, if not aloud, "My God, how much does that person eat?" While the question of caloric intake is a key factor, it is also well recognized, well known, and reasonably well understood.

The evidence does not support that kind of familiarity with the role that water plays. For example, it is not well understood that water retention has a dependent relationship with the amount of **sodium** (as from **salt**!) in the system. **For water to be held by the body, it needs sodium (as in table salt!). The greater the sodium intake, the greater the amount of water the body will retain.** In illustrating this rule, I have often remarked to clients and/or audiences that "bodies of water are larger than bodies of land!" This seems to help focus their attention on water's relationship to weight.

In an era where (pure drinking) water has become a major revenue-generating industry, public sensitivity becomes dulled to the 'down side' of water consumption (as has been our sensitivities to families living on city streets as "the homeless!"). We "see" homeless people everywhere: in village and hamlet, at home and abroad. So, it is with individuals carrying and drinking "bottled water." They are everywhere!

As in some games of competition, there is a rule that where there is "no harm," there is "no foul!" Where water is consumed, without being retained (insufficient sodium in the system), there is little or "no harm" done by the consumption of the pure drinking water (in relation to weight control).

The Salt/Sodium Factor

However, where an overweight body is concerned, there is already possible evidence that this organism has retained water, significantly adding to the overall weight or poundage. This situation implies, therefore, that <u>a lot of salt is being consumed</u>, as salt is the principal source of sodium in our bodies.

Now, it is possible with the water-sodium paradigm to calculate—more or less—the exact ratio of sodium (salt consumption) required to retain "x" amount of water; and this ratio can then be shown to directly correlate to weight gain, pound-per-pound. Such mathematical exercise is better given to one more proficient in such calculations than this writer; but, nonetheless, the principle is clear. And, it does meet the "common sense test" and is consistent with our "cause and effect" premise. Sodium-connected water retention is a major factor in the obesity of many individuals, and in those who are "just overweight."

It is also worthy of note that individuals who are not obese, but still are overweight, must seriously look—first—at their consumption of sodium (through various and sundry salt-laden foods, and from salt used both in food preparation and in table consumption of food).

Nor is it unusual to see overweight individuals "frequently" drinking water (from a vessel 'parked' nearby). This "constant' intake of water is in violation of the Natural Hygiene admonition, according to Drs. T. C. Fry, Herbert M. Shelton, John H. Tilden, V. V. Vetrano, Harvey Diamond, and others, that we should drink pure water (distilled) "only when thirsty."

As with many of the "rules" we hear, or advertisers' themes we see in billboards, on television, or read in print, very often "the real truth" may not surface in what we are led to believe. For example, the admonition that we should drink "eight to ten glasses of water each day" is less than correct advice! Depending upon a number of factors, such as eating style, size, weight, condition, location, activities, temperature, etc., such advice is in possible conflict with teachings of the proven and highly reliable science of natural hygiene.

A large part of the "smoke screen" of advertisements and catchy phrases is that they are designed to sell products (and services), not to assist us in managing our individual wellness programs. Another example is "Milk makes a body strong." Nothing could be farther from the truth, especially since we are speaking of humans! Milk makes a body gain weight (rapidly, as with animals on the savanna plains, which must grow rapidly to keep up with the herd and escape predators!). "2%" and other varieties of milk are like "diet sodas." They are all illusions!

Of course, with young seals, whales, elephants, rhinos, and other large mammals there is increased strength, as the body grows bigger. But, the "strength" illusion in cows' milk ads is the distortion, the 'slight of hand,' the falsification. Little birds, for example, that drink no milk, also grow stronger within hours of their births; and so it is with many other creatures. Without milk, it would be impossible for an elephant to gain its mass, or for a whale to do so—and numerous other mammals—in so short a time frame. Dairy products also put weight on humans.

The point here is that those "who care about wellness" (Anderson, 1986) and want to know what is truth from what is fiction, must re-examine what they believe, hear, read, and see in relation to their managing a successful wellness effort that can deliver them from the disadvantages of overweight, obesity, and from ill health associated with this entire issue. Libraries do house correct information; and there are other sources, including "The Internet."

So, let me repeat: the water-sodium construct is a major contributor to weight gain, overweight, and obesity. It is a subtle factor because it has been so clearly over-looked. The consumption of salt (sodium) clearly contributes to the failures of diet programs, and of wellness and fitness regimens because salt intake is left unchecked, unnoticed, or unconsidered for the vital role the water-salt factor plays in the problems of weight, organ failure, and overall ill health.

Sources of Sodium (Salt)

Before reviewing the food or calorie connection to weight gain, overweight and obesity, let us look briefly at some of the more subtle sources of sodium intake. We do this—please remember—because sodium is the critical requirement for the body to "demand" and retain water. Without the sodium (salt) the body would simply dispose of the excess water, and there would be none left to add weight or other body damage.

Almost all foods identified in the S.A.D. (Standard American Diet) are salt-laden. They run the gamut—from children's cereals to "organic popcorn." **Salt** is a principal component in the making of ice cream; it is in most varieties of chips, sauces, and dairy products. Many "soft drinks" and other beverages contain salt. The flesh foods (chicken, fish, beef, pork, turkey, game, etc.) industry is nearly absolutely dependent upon salt to sell and market their flesh food products. For, who among you will eat meat products without salt? Restaurants all over the world, and housewives in their kitchens have a strong bond with salt as a necessary element in cooking and preparing their foods. Even so-called dessert foods tend to include a significant amount of salt. Not only is salt an embalming substance (perhaps better known for "smoking" and "curing" beef, ham, fish, pork, turkey, and other flesh foods), it is, perhaps, the most commonly associated element in the human food chain.

We are already quite familiar with the connections between salt and high blood pressure, heart disease, diabetes, stroke, and many highly recognized ailments, including cancers and *immune-deficient conditions*. Like its look-a-like, and equally destructive 'cousin' (sugar), salt and sugar could be called "silent or invisible killers." Both claim more lives annually than do cocaine, "AIDS," cancers, and military wars throughout history! Yet, from a purely natural hygiene perspective, neither sugar nor salt kills people. Dr. V. V. Vetrano advises that, "People die from enervation, resulting from toxemia enhanced by the ingestion of sugars and salts."

It is salt, however, not sugar that is the culprit in holding water in the system. According to Dr. Vetrano, "Drinking excess water overworks the kidneys, just as does eating table salt. There are numerous physiologic processes that are required to maintain the *sodium and water* balance. The endocrine glands and other organs must do extra work to maintain the proper volume of the blood, and for normal sodium, calcium and water balance. So," she concludes, "it is enervating to drink more water than needed, but the body finds it necessary if people are **salt addicts**. Salt is a stimulant and it enervates. Hence, it is an enervator." The ultimate manifestation is "a crisis of toxemia," as John H. Tilden, MD declared disease to be. It is what leads to what the world knows as a variety of disease conditions commonly called cancers.

Cancers in Children

In a sense, all forms of cancer have their genesis in the consumption of compounds of salt. And, there are many forms of salt that are consumed from the human food chain. Table salt—like white sugar—is just the most harmful or ultimately, perhaps, the most deadly! In children, for example, it is possible to establish beyond a reasonable doubt that it is *the intake of white sugar and of white salt that eventually leads to cancer as the number one killer of our children!* **For advertisers and parents to continue to ignore this vital connection is tantamount to what Dr. Bernard Jensen has referred to as "a criminal act," a crime against children.** Nor can parents continue to be "excused," either because they were not properly taught (either in school or in their mothers' kitchens) or because they are deceived, misled, and "pressured" by advertisers and by agencies (social and governmental).

If governments do not step in to protect the children (perhaps not a most popular notion!), then conceivably churches, religious groups, and charitable organizations will move more into this vacuum. They could teach or "preach a gospel of wellness" and use this and similar volumes as the "curriculum" for a truly safe and sane wellness program that will prevent overweight, obesity, ill health, and cancer deaths, among children as well as among adults.

I have written in the past—especially when it comes to famines in "developing countries"—that we should look, first, to the water people drink. In an interview in Lagos, Nigeria, with the Minister of Health, The Honorable Prof. Ransome-Kuti, this writer urged: "If you purify Nigeria's drinking water, the incidents of sickness and disease will drop 90%!" (of course, assuming that people are well fed on healthy foods). In the years since that interview (1992), the drinking water industry in Nigeria has grown exponentially! Though the data are not presently available to this writer, I believe statistics will support the conclusion that there does exist a corresponding decline in the number and types of sickness and disease conditions treated or otherwise reported during the same period (1992-2001). "But," adds Dr. Vetrano, "what about the chemicals used to treat water? Chorine and its by products have been studied and found guilty of increasing the risk of bladder and rectal cancer."

Calories and Weight Control

We are all familiar with "the calorie connection" to weight gain, overweight, and obesity. But, again, what we "see" is <u>not</u> what the reality is. We look at calories and attribute to them the responsibility or "credit" for our "putting on the pounds." Herein lies the "slight of hand" we have constantly referred to in this volume. What we see is not what we get, to put it plainly.

So, let us review the role of calories from a different perspective. Let us ask a different type of question. For example, if you weigh 400 pounds (or any weight, really), what number of calories will you require daily **to not lose** any of your 400lbs?

In other words, since we all have been taught that calories add weight to our bodies (so, we watch out for those high calorie foods!), it is just as fair for us to examine the "cause and effect" rule that: failing to consume "x" numbers of calories will result in a reduction or loss in weight (for that particular day, or period of time). Again, a college algebra student can easily calculate these co-factors; but, that is not our task here.

Calorie intake keeps weight on. We want to establish in the literature—for all time—that in order to maintain body weight at a certain level, it is probable that such body must take in a 'corresponding' number of calories per day—without exception!

Of course, we say 'without exception' to re-establish our point (in as much as we have already looked at the water-salt connection to weight gain, overweight, obesity, and ill health): *since the intake of calories causes us to put on pounds, the intake of "an equivalent amount" of calories is required to maintain that same weight.* It has been many years since I excelled in high school geometry (even beating my teacher, who solved a geometry problem in twelve steps that I solved in eight!). But, I believe still that "things equal to the same thing are equal to each other."

If calories add weight, calories are required to sustain weight. Prof. Peter Duesberg proved this corollary for the National Health Institute when his sponsored research study to "prove HIV caused AIDS" produced an unexpected and unacceptable result! Only 50% of AIDS victims tested positive for "HIV." Therefore, Prof. Duesberg rightly concluded, "HIV does not and cannot cause AIDS…For an agent to be 'causal' that agent must always be present" (not just in only half the instances!). That conclusion was not what the Establishment wanted back from this noted and (formerly) highly respected researcher within the scientific community!

So, we must conclude that if overweight individuals fail to consume daily calories sufficient to sustain their overweight, then they would lose weight! Put differently, when individuals fail to lose weight despite the "diet" or weight-loss program they employ, it is because they are still consuming the calories (or water weight) to sustain their undesired weight levels. The same goes for water retention. If less water (sodium) was consumed, less water weight would be held, and the individual would lose some weight that day, or during any specified period of time. Over her many years as a fasting expert, Dr. Vetrano states, "I have seen obese individuals lose as much as 15 pounds on the first day of a fast. They lose less after that. There is a lot of water stored in fatty tissue. The first few days of fasting these individuals are seldom thirsty."

U.S. Congresswoman Maxine Waters has come to be associated with the expression, "No justice, no peace!" a cry of outrage during the civil disturbances that followed the acquittal of the twenty-five officers in the infamous Rodney King beating trial in Los Angeles in 1992. That incident was viewed by television audiences around the world; but, the jury concluded, "These officers were just defending themselves." More recently, the Rev. Al Sharpton, the "self-proclaimed successor" to the Rev. Jesse Jackson, has championed the phrase, "No justice, No peace!" and employed it in his support of Puerto Rican citizens protesting the high rate of sickness, disease, and cancer in people impacted by military chemical activities around the military base. This is not about who was first to use the phrase; it is rather just an illustration of the "cause and effect" theme that is fundamental to all concepts and hypotheses discussed in this volume. And, I think we have made our points.

A Final Word on Water Weight

As a final word on the water weight issue, let me just say this: if you or anyone you communicate with find it unreasonable to associate water retention with weight gain, overweight, and obesity, you will have to identify your own controlling factor or factors. For, while there is some relationship between not chewing food very well before swallowing; between overeating; between calorie intake; between animal protein (oils, fats, etc.) and weight gain, none of these except, perhaps, **calorie intake**, will be found to rival water retention as a critical factor in weight gain, over weight, obesity, ill health, and the onset of cancer—especially in children!

Dr. Vetrano further explains the construct, thusly: "Let me point out that water is not a true gain in weight as is fat, because the water is eliminated very quickly when fasting and when one quits eating **salt and spices**, and other tissue irritants. At most, there could be not much more water weight than 15-20 pounds."

"Nevertheless," she continues, "when fasting and the body begins to metabolize fat or energy, water is a bi-product of the breakdown process. This is because fat contains a lot of hydrogen."

These are, perhaps, "radical" ideas. If they are, that could be good. If they are hypotheses that are unreasonable, they will fail "the common sense test," and no one will be deceived. A practical verification study (that anyone can conduct) is to somehow measure the daily salt and water intake of extremely overweight individuals. In a friendly, helpful, and supportive environment, such a study would represent a "win-win" situation for all concerned. And, unless there is a reason the truth should not be known, those involved shall have to be the judges, and will bear the ultimate responsibility for their decisions.

As for this writer, and others who have contributed so much to this volume, you are urged to discard anything herein that comes up short when it is judged alongside that which makes common sense. For, in all we see in Nature or know through our God-given instincts, nothing should become a guide for our lives unless it passes "the common sense test" or is otherwise "based in Faith," as the Rev. Joyce Bowie-Guillory of Atlanta, Georgia would espouse.

International and Ethnic Foods

The eating styles and patterns of peoples around the world are, of course, more related to disease conditions among them than to weight gain, overweight, and obesity *per se*. For example, high fat, high sugar consumption of pastries in India contributes significantly to the country's high percentage of diabetes. As a "vegetarian" country, one would expect India's overweight and allied health problems to be less than for meat-eating countries; but, it is not necessarily the case.

Taiwan, as an affluent nation, is a prime example of a country that tends to be "over fed, overweight, and overly subjected to the ills of a high-fat, high-protein, and highly diseased culture." There was a time when the "Made in Taiwan" label was attached to almost any consumer product one handled. The resulting wealth and "cultural exchange" led to changes in eating styles, with more American "fast food" logo's dotting the Taiwan skyline.

Today, "Made in China" seems to have become the "favorite nation" for the production of consumer goods for the American market. This two-way cooperation will graduate into measurable differences in weight and disease issues within the Chinese culture. The pattern will not be so different from what happened in Japan, when the world was privy to the "Made in Japan" labels. Heart disease—today a significant concern in Japan—was virtually unknown during the early years after World War II.

Here at home, the "soul food" eating style of African Americans (Washitaw or the Indigenous people of "the Americas") is directly related to (is the "cause" of) the "grim" health statistics frequently reported in the press, in research papers, and in grant proposals. Soul food has all the negatives (and a number of positives as well)! It is highly cooked; highly salted; highly animal protein; highly seasoned; high in fat; high in cholesterol; high in starch; high in white sugar; high in oil (grease, even lard); and from a Natural Hygiene perspective, soul food is high in chemical by-products (poisons) produced when these elements are subjected to extreme heat, as in cooking.

The positive features of the collard and cabbage family of greens (as a control for so-called 'sickle cell anemia') along with yam, apricot, broccoli, and baby spinach, notwithstanding, soul food must be charged with the propensity for overweight among these Washitaw, indigenous people (now referred to as African Americans, Indian Americans, and by other names).

In all these "ethnic foods," the common elements are the marriages between sodium and water, animal protein and putrefaction, toxemia and enervation, and consequently lead to the suffering, reduced quality of life, and premature death from the host of disease conditions we have looked at time and again: diabetes, heart disease, prostate and other cancers, stroke, MS, high blood pressure or hypertension, sickle cell anemia and a variety of so-called 'anemia' (early-stage blood cancer or blood toxemia), and on the listing could go.

Time and space have been given to an extended discussion of the "ethnic foods connection" to weight gain, overweight, and disease conditions for two primary reasons: 1) Individuals still do not see—or are too irrefutably "programmed" to acknowledge—the relationship between what they eat (the "cause") and the disease conditions they suffer (the "effect"), <u>as a class of people</u>. 2) Failing to "see" or understand what causes their problems, they remain "victims" of their own blindness, and become "funding sources" for the medical establishment, which welcomes their economic contributions to the Establishment's "bottom line."

From a moralistic perspective, the "tragedy" in the above picture is likewise twofold: a) The refusal or inability to "break with" traditional eating styles ("soul" or ethnic foods might be good for the soul, but they are bad for health!) provides the platform for all the varieties of disease conditions suffered by "ethnic eaters." And, unless the eating patterns improve, the negative disease statistics will also <u>not</u> improve. And, (b) All of the problems—diabetes, heart disease, stroke, high blood pressure, hypertension, prostate cancer, bladder cancer, kidney failure, liver failure, arthritis, asthma, "sickle cell anemia," and other so-called 'ethnic diseases'—can be, literally, brought under control 'over night.'

"Early screening, early detection, early diagnosis, early treatment" are more "smoke screens." For, as T. C. Fry said years ago, "Disease will not occur if its cause is not engaged." These "screenings" give false hope, and are deceptive; they are more "slight of hand." What's more medical tests are estimated to make up 90% of the physician's income! Changing how you eat, drink, exercise, and rest will change how you suffer—or not suffer! Individuals are the masters of their fates, imbued by their Creator with "free will." The human legacy is one that supports love, truth, peace, freedom, and justice among all the peoples of this earth.

Disease is, rather, a consequence of poor choices. Weight gain, overweight, and obesity are but "reminders" in our lives that we have not exercised the better options available to us. As a matter of common sense, we should not expect professionals who earn their envied lifestyles from our "preferred blindness" and dependency upon them—to surrender this monetary advantage by beating us over the head with admonitions that would not require our visits to their offices and facilities. Would you bite the hand that feeds you?

Chapter Sixteen

'Wellness Menopause'

We are generally familiar with the term "menopause." We know that it relates to a biological process in women, which seems to occur between the ages of forty-five and fifty-five. It is the culmination, actually, of a much longer set of dynamics, which began back at the onset of puberty when the young girl experienced her first menstruation. That is Nature's way of signaling that the female of the species is now ready for procreation. There are signals of 'menopause' in the male of the species as well; however, our focus will exclude him for the moment.

The American Heritage Dictionary (1974) gives this definition of <u>menopause</u>: *The period of cessation of menstruation, occurring usually between the ages of 45 and 50*; <u>menstruation</u> as *The process or an instance of discharging the menses*; and <u>menses</u> as <u>*blood and dead cell debris*</u> *discharged from the uterus through the vagina by adult women at approximately monthly intervals between puberty and menopause*. These definitions take us full cycle, from beginning to end.

But, many women will readily admit that for them, menopause represented not just an 'ending,' but rather a worrisome and troubling 'beginning.' An entire sub-industry has developed around "what many women need <u>after menopause</u>!" Whether or not I think such marketing of services and products is totally justified is not the focus for now, and would be a distraction for me to present any counter argument. Suffice it to say that as my central point is developed, the reader will have no trouble ascertaining what my views are on the above subject.

Nature is extremely consistent in what She does; and She does the *same* thing in many different ways and at various levels throughout Creation, animate and inanimate. So, let us take another look at our definition of menses. In particular, we note that what is thrown off by the body is "blood and dead cell debris." About blood we know that it is not only the largest body organ, but that it is also the body's major "transport system." So, naturally, we can expect such "dead cells and debris" to be carried by the blood stream and expelled according to Nature's preordination. Of course, this entails the passing of some very used or special purpose blood as well.

Dr. T. C. Fry has stated elsewhere in this volume that the human organism experiences the death of trillions of cells daily; that this dead cell matter is also very deadly, if not expelled. And this is true for men as well as for women. In fact, Dr. Fry contends that it is the very accumulation of internal poisons, which include "dead cell debris" that is the basis of most disease conditions in human beings. Dr. John H. Tilden, in advance of Dr. Fry's pronouncement, declared that dis-ease in the human organism represents "a crisis of toxemia." Dr. Herbert M. Shelton spent most of his life researching, writing and confirming his notion that "all diseases are the same disease."

What are these Natural Hygiene giants saying, really? My summation is this: *All un-expelled substances within the organism, whether generic to the organism or foreign, are toxic and over time 'this stuff' produces the 'symptoms' commonly referred to as "diseases."* Put another way, stuff turns into garbage; and *garbage in equals garbage out.*

This proposition seems simple enough; in fact, it seems too simple. And because it is so uncomplicated and logical, this very truth undercuts much of what we have been taught about diseases—especially about "causes and cures." If what we have said above is as true as it is simple, one might ask: "Where, in the end, will researching and testing for cures lead us, if not right back to 'actions which prevent the onset of symptoms' in the first instance?" All animal laboratory experimenting, and work on human cadavers become suspect (another "slight of hand" or magic trick)!

Given the proven reliability of our "cause and effect" structure, individuals "who care about wellness" can regain power over their lives. **Nothing robs an individual of his or her freedom more quickly than the instruction: "Take off all your clothes; the doctor will be with you in a moment."** Your voluntary submission, supported by how your parents raised you, and by all the things you have been 'taught' about *the nature and purpose of disease* left you little or no alternative but to do as you were told. In your mind—as was in my own mind for years—the alternative could lead to "my untimely death." So, understandably much of your 'obedience' is generated by fear; and sustained fear is a form of enslavement. Sustained fear—fear nurtured by false constructs and misinformation—goes far beyond our natural instincts of "fight or flight."

The simplicity of what my gurus taught is emancipating! For more than fifteen years, now, I have been free! I feel like I am in control of my life—of my health, of my well being, of my happiness, of my future, and of my death. I no longer concern myself with "coming down with some catastrophic disease." I have an understanding of how the organism works—of what causes it to be at dis-ease or out of balance, and what brings it back into balance. I have no "family doctor" and I carry no "health insurance" (but, I do carry "accident insurance," for both injury and death). But, disease symptoms and/or conditions are never "accidental." **Disease is like murder: there is always traceable cause.**

When murders go unsolved, it is because those charged with solving the murders are looking in the wrong places, seeing the wrong "clues," misreading the evidence, thrown off by their own perceptions, or a combination of these and other factors. The point has been made, for example, about the trillions of dollars spent on cancer research: "You cannot find rabbits at the tops of trees." Thus, no "cure" for cancer in forty years, despite the billions of dollars spent on "research," and all the (false) "hope" entertained by the gullible public. Had individuals been told the truth, many would still be alive; and the quality of many other lives would have improved drastically. All of this might have happened without spending "one dollar" on cancer research!

The simple truth that Shelton, Tilden, Fry and others continue to put before us is cause for excitement! I have been passionate about sharing my excitement since my own "light bulb moment" (Thanks, Oprah for the phrase!) in 1986! So grateful I am for the freedom I feel that I cannot stop trying to find different ways to tell the world this simple story: You do not have to be sick; you do not have to "anticipate" degenerative diseases later in life; and you do not have to surrender your life and assets to an army of "practicing professionals" who tell you over and over and over: "We have no cure; but, let's try this."

Nor am I unrealistic. I am quite aware that children are brought up by parents who traumatize daily whether the child or children will "survive to become healthy adults." I also know how confused parents are kept—from the day the child is brought home from the hospital to the time of inoculations to first enter school. I am aware what public agencies demand; and how other parents are deceived, threatened and frightened as well. I am not here arguing with these constructs, even though you have no problem sensing my discontent.

What I more want to focus on is another simple fact that we all are aware of: <u>information is power</u>. But, for this power to be positive and constructive, it must be based upon reliable information. It has to emanate from truth; and for a thing to be true it must meet 'the common sense test.' It cannot be true for you and for me if it is knowable only to the research scientist or to the Rhodes scholar.

The point here is that I liberated myself my accessing ***reliable information*** that held up under the test of common sense; and I have continued to verify and re-verify my perceptions from the writings and teachings of authors listed in this volume and many who are not listed, and by some who do not publish. I am convinced that you, too, can have a choice.

Opting for Liberation

The road to liberation is short or long depending upon your own motivation, commitment and implementation of "actions that prevent the occurrence of disease conditions in the first place." The necessary—and correct—information is abundantly available. Of this you can be certain. But, there is so much incorrect information flooding the market it is easy to be "doubtful, confused, frustrated, or even resentful" that 'a clear picture' of the simple truth is not more available. This, you can do something about.

What I strongly recommend is following Nature's example. Consider the period of our childhood, teen years, early adulthood and maturity as the period during which our organisms 'automatically' expelled "toxins and dead cell debris" (remember pimples, acne, 'the common cold,' flu and even 'childhood diseases?'). Consider this: children who received no animal products, including dairy, or inoculations "almost never came down with any of the so-called childhood diseases." Children who are not consumers of "the average" amounts of sugars (from candy, bread, cake, ice cream, cookies, soft drinks, popular cereals, and other concentrated 'foods') grow up much less hard to manage, and become adults who seldom experience Alzhimers, diabetes, mental illness, heart disease, stroke; and, as children, escape their number one killer—cancer (albeit, by the several names it is given when it kills the young!).

Am I suggesting there is a relationship between diets and diseases? You bet I am! But, what is diet, really? As a former elementary, secondary and adult school teacher, counselor and administrator; and, as a former college lecturer, university supervisor of student-teachers, professor and university administrator, I will define a person's diet just as I used to define a school's curriculum (Revolutionary Urban Teaching, Anderson, 1973): *It is everything that is experienced by the student in the name of schooling.* That means the school's curriculum begins at the home, follows children to school, in school, in the name of school, and back home (with all its varied dynamics). This is what the school's true curriculum is. What a child consumes is his or her diet (including violent video games, soft drinks, vulgar language, fast and junk foods, sweets, and even molestation or abuse). These produce chemicals within the organism; and some of this stuff leads to toxicity, the foundation for cancers. Do you know how much fear or anxiety your child endures on a daily basis?

A person's diet, then, is much more than the food and beverage consumed. It is also the air one breathes; the water one drinks; the beliefs one holds dear; the fears; the joys; the anxieties; the longings; the disappointments; the love and the hate; sunshine and the warmth; sense of protection; security; hope for a reasonable future; and many other "consumables" are the individual's *diet*. One's diet should involve exercise, rest, adequate sleep, frequent bowel elimination, peaceful feeding, tranquility and normal stress.

So, once again, what is disease? Disease a direct result of accumulated toxins and dead cell debris that was not expelled from the organism in a timely manner. Why—if it is so simple, and we can know this—why is this deadly stuff not expelled in a timely manner? The question is good and simple; so is the answer: because, as Spike Lee, the movie producer, put it, individuals do not "do the right thing(s)." The proof of this is that many among us often spend large sums of money before realizing they can help themselves—and they do! Entertainers, some athletes, professional people, poor people, people in "developing countries," Natural Hygienists, wholistic practitioners, and others not prone to consuming large amounts of animal products, drugs and herbs often are astonishing with their great looks and good health! So, we do have plenty of 'role models' and the benefits are quite free of "confusion."

Not everyone wants to be healthy. Yes, this is true. Being healthy limits the kind of actions one can take, on the one hand; and, it requires one to take certain regular actions, on the other hand. Remember, the reliable natural paradigm—"cause and effect?" People seem to prefer believing what is not true, "because that is how I was raised!" One Beverly Hills client who wanted to lose weight and improve a long-time skin condition responded this way when I suggested she might cut out the consumption of animal products for some time: "What! Give up eating steaks?" I suggested she return when she was truly concerned about her wellness. Respecting, if you will, an adult's God-given right to opt for a healthier or less healthier life experience is why my first book in this field was entitled, *Helping Hand: 8-Day Diet Programs* ***for People Who Care about Wellness.*** People do have the God-Given Right to <u>not</u> care.

Let us assume that, for now, you are an individual who has decided you want to experience and possess many of the benefits alluded to in the previous paragraphs, and throughout this book, really! What should you do—specifically? You should initiate a **wellness menopause,** or a basic change in the way you eat, drink, exercise and rest. I will tell you how to do this.

First, avail yourself of reliable information. Many books are available. Perhaps the best known in recent years is Harvey and Marilyn Diamond's blockbuster bestseller, *Fit for Life.* This single volume changed the way millions of peoples worldwide considered their personal options for being well and maintaining optimum health. Harvey and Marilyn were also students of our common guru, T. C. Fry who, himself was a student of Dr. Herbert M. Shelton, considered "the father of Natural Hygiene." Dr. Shelton defined 'Natural Hygiene' as "that system of biology which focuses on the natural requirements of the human organism," which lead to and maintain optimum well being for the organism.

Second, emancipate yourself from adherence to "superstition, propaganda, orchestrated fear, and illogical constructs." There are many examples of these. It is not the "chicken soup" grandma gave us that helped us recover (return to balance); it was, instead, the act of providing little or no food—fasting—as the true remedy. That is how Nature "treats" organic imbalance (disease symptoms). Take a quick 'mental journey' to the savannas of East Africa. Behold the thousands of huge animals, and not one veterinarian doctor! Now sprint back to your own quarters; and, if you are a pet owner, answer this question: How do you know when your pet is not well? That is it: Your pet refuses all offers of food! Guess what? So do infants! With animals and babies, Nature is still in control. Adult humans are different; God gave them freewill! Humans believe that the number 13 and walking under a ladder are bad luck; but, they do not think that of consuming alcohol and drugs, especially "designer drugs" like cocaine (the single-most "cause" of the effect generally known as "HIV-AIDS!"). It is more comfortable believing what is not true: that "unsafe sex" or body fluids or even more mystical, "a virus" is the cause. And why not believe the lie? After all, $2 million dollar a year news readers remind us everyday of "HIV, the virus that causes AIDS." How convenient for—and protective of—the drug industry, both the legal and the illegal arms of that super wealthy industrial complex that actually owns the major media outlets! Our confusion and misinformation are critical to the vulgar success of the pharmaceutical/chemical industry. We have finally exposed and are holding accountable the tobacco industry; when will we expose and hold accountable the pharmaceutical/chemical bandits?

Thirdly, put the information gathered to the "common sense test." In other words, do all you can to 'challenge' the information. For example, T. C. Fry's writings decry all medications as "poisons." Challenge this notion by asking your doctor or pharmacist: "Are there any known drugs that do not have 'side effects?'" Any "effect" is a consequence, a result (usually negative) that did not exist before. A broken leg is a consequence of trauma; a cavity is the consequence of acidity, putrefaction, fermentation and 'corrosive' actions in the warmth of the mouth; and, as we have stated before, murder is the effect (the killer or killers are the cause). John Harris, a wholistic seminar sponsor, was correct when he said, so prophetically: "If you keep on doing what you've been doing, you will keep on getting what you've been getting!"

Fourthly, you must *decide* "it is time to make a change in how I eat, drink, exercise and rest." This decision is extremely important. When clients come to me, or call up on the telephone wanting to know, for example, should they undertake a fast, my first question is: "Why do you want to go on a fast?" What I listen for is a substantive reason. What I have gotten too often is: "I want to lose about ten pounds so I will fit better in my new dress for a special party coming up." Or, a rather obese gentleman proclaimed, "I need to lose about 70 pounds." One middle-aged office manager "just felt bloated." Your decision must come from a personal commitment to take charge of your life. At least, to begin taking charge is the second most important reason for electing to modify how you eat and live. Perhaps the most important reason is having come to the realization that *you do have a choice.*

Fifth, you must systematically and religiously implement the correct consumptive behaviors into your daily living routine. If you have ever been a smoker and quit, you know how 'strict' you had to be in not tolerating the presence of cigarette smoke in your private space. No matter where you were, or who might be the offender, you knew you just had to separate yourself from the bad environment of the cigarette smoke. Likewise, when you begin implementing the recommended actions into your wellness regime, no matter who attempts to dissuade you, you must be steadfast. Nor is it necessary to be either offensive or apologetic. You only need to be committed, to yourself, to your new goal, to the anticipation of the wonderful benefits in store for you. For once you have experienced a few of these great and wonderful changes in your life, then and only then can you share your new knowledge, experience and joy with others.

Lastly, you must study by researching, reading, listening, learning, and practicing what Natural Hygiene preaches. In this on-going process you will be able to verify and re-verify what you thought you learned earlier. This is important because you are taking control of your own life, and by possible influence, the lives of others who want to be like you. There is a story that might illustrate the importance of verification and re-verification. A man who had practiced Natural Hygiene for years began to suffer weakening illness. He was seen by Hygienic physicians and even contacted allopathic physicians. In the end the man's condition worsen and he died. His demise was most alarming because everyone considered him a model practitioner of the most recommended lifestyle actions. Quite by accident, someone very dear to the man came across a major principle by which the deceased man had lived. In reviewing the principle, the friend discovered *a typographical error.* In a critical passage, the word "not" had been omitted; and all those years, the dead man had been doing just the opposite of what the literature encouraged. I cannot say whether this simple story is a true story; but I repeat it here for the point that it makes. **Many words sound the same, but have different meanings; many statements can be interpreted quite differently. And, sometimes, omissions or additions are made. Uncorrected, these could send followers down the wrong path. By constantly re-verifying you eventually eliminate such regretful errors.**

No "take charge wellness program" can deliver all you would want without having a fasting dimension. We have already shown that "hygienic fasting" is Nature's preferred remedy for recapturing organic balance. We alluded to animals and babies not accepting food when they were feeling "out of balance." So critical is the subject of fasting I have decided to devote an entire chapter to the subject. That discussion will follow.

When to Change Bad Diet Habits

Before leaving the discussion of undergoing a "wellness menopause," I want to re-emphasize a few points. Routinely, every adult (females included) should decide at an early age to stop the unhealthy practices in their lifestyles. What age that might be, of course, depends upon the individual. For me, that time came when looking down towards the floor, I could see neither my feet nor my genitals!

And, there were other indications that I might need to change my consumptive behavior. Sex, a long-time favorite, was becoming less and less 'attractive.' On the basketball court, it was hard to convince my son that I had ever played the game, either in college or in high school. In the business world I found myself losing my competitive edge; my mind was less sharp, and not as quick. Most troubling was that my "photographic memory" was increasingly unable to reproduce those clear images of earlier years. I knew something was going in the wrong direction.

Individuals will experience a variety of telltale indications that "there might be a potential problem developing." Where there is no pain associated with the symptom (weight gain, for example) people tend to accept the condition as a 'natural' consequence of growing older. Many people begin to notice skin discoloration, or an acne-type condition. Great numbers around the world find themselves, too frequently, combating "the common cold" or "malaria" or some other familiarly-named symptom. Perhaps the most common pain producing indication is the stiffening of the joints as in arthritis.

As incredible as it may seem, more than half the people in Western society already are well on their way toward the onset of heart disease and cancer by the age of twenty! Many school children, cancer's biggest victims, cannot pass the simplest of fitness tests, wrote T.C. Fry in 1974. I once demonstrated push-ups to an eight-year-old grand-nephew Marcus, then challenged him to see how many he could do. The lad was obviously overweight; his mind told him he could outdo his "old uncle." I will always remember the shocked look on his face, and the disappointment in his body language, when he could not push his own weight from the floor a single time!

These patterns or "signs of the onset of disease conditions" are really indications of improper living—centered, primarily, on what, if not how, we consume. The preponderance of the evidence is clear: our Standard American Diet (SAD), which includes wrong foods as well as too little exercise and other human essentials, is what brings about pain, suffering, and a reduction in the quality of life, much too early in life.

I lost my first wife to cancer—after 36 years and 3 months of 'holy bliss.' Her eating habits were animal-based and she was not athletic. She believed in taking vitamins and prescription drugs. I am just the opposite. During the four years of her ordeal, I dropped everything to be with her—night and day. During the first two years, we traveled to all the places we used to enjoy together. During the last two, I observed many correlations; and thought much about what I saw.

She had gone 'into remission' when she accepted mostly fruits, vegetables, nuts and seeds—raw and organically grown—for her meals; and her distress soon returned when she demanded animal products and sweets. Of course, there were other factors. My point is simply this: the notion of 'cause and effect' seems abstract until you watch someone you love slowly die from a condition that could have been prevented had food consuming behaviors changed earlier, and were maintained later.

I am convinced that cancer and diet, like "HIV-AIDS" and drugs are as related as females are to giving birth! The 'cause and effect' construct casts such a light, no wonder it seems 'blinding.' There is little more than a funeral parlor industry surrounding "natural death," while cancer and "HIV-AIDS" are the world's best "health care" money makers (excluding the vast incomes from performing tests!). A cynic benefactor might well put forth this argument: "People are going to die anyway; why just let it happen without capitalizing on their dying?" I often wished the pain and sorrow of grieving families was enough to touch the medical establishment! But, how can it?

I have seen first hand the high cost of "medical services." I am not impressed! I watched daily as my mother lay dying in her hospital bed—over a three-week period. Among her eight living children, at least two were with her around the clock. She had no 'operations' or 'procedures' and very little else; but, upon her death, from "heart failure," the family was presented with a medical bill of $97,236.81—more than $20,000 of which was listed as "drugs." Though I never saw all of the billings for my wife's nearly two years of intense services, I am certain her insurance was billed more than $1,000,000.00!

Many sensitive issues are raised when it comes to the high cost of medical services, and the lack of correlation between money spent and patient recovery. So, I will leave this issue and return to where you and I can remain "in control." By initiating our own "change of life (style)" or wellness menopause, we substantially stop poisoning ourselves into premature pain, suffering and death. As my late guru, mentor, co-author, and friend, T. C. Fry, has articulated so often, we cannot arrive at health through the ritual or practice of consuming poisons, whether in our food chain or by "taking poisons euphemistically called medicines."

Accumulated "Stuff" Poisons the Organism

When internal toxicity—mostly from foods, drugs, and memories—has accumulated so rapidly as to bring about disease conditions, like cancer, at an early age (35-55), it is referred to as "catastrophic disease." This implies that the person suffers from an unexpected, unusual set of circumstances (that are not, by the way, related at all to the person's historic diet or consumption and retention experience). Of course, such notion is pure deception, as we have shown over and over.

We see how deceptive such perception is when we look at the plight of our elders, whom we 'expect' to come down with stuff at their ages! Truth of the matter is that the onset of disease symptoms is more related to non-eliminated toxic build-up than it is to individual age. A healthy, active senior is so because unwanted stuff, dangerous internal poisons, have been regularly and routinely eliminated, for the most part, through the actions that support wellness. Were it not so the older person would not be healthy at his or her attained age. Don't forget, many children don't make it out of childhood!

Realistically, as most of us witness in our everyday lives, our seniors—but less often "young seniors," who look and act fit—either are 'seized' by some crippling condition, or they face some terrifying diagnosis, sooner or later. In either case, the prognosis is not good. Experience shows that such older persons have a "declining life expectancy" to look forward to. Quality of life becomes increasingly dependent upon others; and, the "high cost of dying" begins to take charge.

In younger persons, paying "whatever it takes" is largely justified or rationalized by the notion that he or she "can be saved," or "is too young to die." Obviously, productive living should be prolonged; but, more critically, it should be protected. Protection is just another way of expressing "prevention." Preventing the later onset of disease conditions requires us to live by the "rules of wellness" (Anderson, 1986).

Isn't it interesting how good people tend 'to encourage' the use of so-called recreational drugs, for example, then later when the users 'pay the Piper,' these same 'good people' will do one of two things: 1) They become advocates, supporters, sponsors, and/or participants in publicized "AIDS walks/runs" for the expressed purpose of "raising money for research, to find a cure in our life time!" How terribly ironic! 2) They make 'heroes' of the abusers who continue to live, and martyr those who die. So, Jimi Hendrix, the great guitar playing composer-producer-band leader, drug addict dies at age 27 (of 'asphyxiation'); and his abusive behavior becomes enshrined in his legacy. What a 'message' such walk/run parades send children!

Where, in such public response, is there the "righteous indignation" that once led our youth gone astray back to a more responsible existence? Better to die young having "it all" than to live in uncertainty? "It" best describes drugs and its accompanying 'benefits.' Drugs are the <u>cause</u>; and, all too often, early death is the <u>effect</u>.

Parents and loved ones, notwithstanding, this is how it goes. People die young from one of three causes: 1) Poisoning, as in internal build-up, or using drugs and/or chemical substances; 2) Trauma, like an auto accident or act of violence; or 3) Imperfection of Nature, as when an organism cannot long endure because of defects at birth (some of which, by the way, stem not from Nature's 'error' but from the activities of the parents, especially of the father, as in the case of drug usage).

At a public lecture I was giving at a Los Angeles International Airport area hotel, I had just given the above 'three causes of death' and offered $100.00 to anyone in the audience who could suggest a "fourth cause of death." I had already 'proven' that no one dies of "disease" (it is not an "entity," but a "description"). After several responses—all of which were shown to fit the already stated categories—about mid-way back, a nine-year-old African American girl raised her hand. I acknowledged her and this is what she said (to the question, 'Can anyone suggest a fourth cause of death?'): "'Cause they want to!" she said. People also die because they 'will' themselves to die.

The audience fell silent. I was also silent. It seemed like minutes as I raced through my 'three causes,' first considering that the act of dying itself must involve one of my stated causes. Then, just as quickly, I outstretched the hand holding the $100 bill, offering it to the nine-year-old winner! The audience applauded with great uproar as I acknowledged there <u>was</u> a psychological dimension, to living and to dying. People do "will themselves to die." Children, long sexually abused by family, sometimes "decide" Heaven is a better place. While in most cases of suicide it is trauma, the number two cause of death, there are a significant number of instances where the individual "just stopped breathing." So, the nine-year-old took home $100; and my audience and I were reminded of an important lesson.

We abhor the deaths of our young, even more so than we do the lifestyle habits that are known to lead to their demise! Candy in Western society is produced, primarily, for children; cancer is the primary killer of children. Is there no relationship? We 'accept' the deaths of young military and law enforcement personnel because they are perceived to have died in our own best interests. We 'excuse' so-called HIV/AIDS and cancer deaths by blaming a "third entity," either a non-existent or irrelevant "virus" or an "incurable human curse," as with heart disease. <u>We ignore "diet" as cause and "death" as effect.</u>

When people are already old, the tendency is to "keep them as comfortable as possible." This is how hospices are run. Nurse Tom Dorsey, as a visiting hospice nurse supervisor once told me, "Good physicians hold to the adage they should 'do no harm.'" He explained such physicians refuse to prescribe more or stronger medications for their patients "because they believe the 'side effects' of these poisons are more life-threatening than the complaints of their patients."

Nurse Tom sees that practice as "a good thing." This writer agrees. Natural Hygiene agrees. More is not, necessarily, better. What is best, however, is living life in a manner that provides for its essential needs, thereby *preventing* such later circumstances. And, for those who ask: "Yes, but at my age—and in my condition—what can I do now?" T. C. Fry's answer still holds: "Stop poisoning yourself." Permit your organism to eliminate already stored poisons. ***Change what you do—how you consume (change your complete "diet")—to make your actions consistent with those that provide the organism with all of its essential needs. This is what this book is all about!***

Education must supplant treatment; faith in the processes and forces of life must take the place of faith in "cure"; confidence in the normal things of life must displace confidence in abnormal things; trust in the laws of life must crowd out trust in vicarious atonements. Only thus can the ages-long frenzied search of "cure" be ended. Only thus can the terrible waste of time, money, energy and mental effort in the search for "cure" cease and all this time, money, energy and effort be re-directed into profitable channels.

- T. C. Fry

Chapter Seventeen

Hygienic Fasting: A Life Saving Action

First, let us explore some preliminary questions and answers to establish a 'foundation' for receiving life-saving information about the method and technique of hygienic or 'organic wellness' fasting.

Question: Will I die if I don't eat for three or four days?

Answer: *People have been known to live for as long as six months without taking in food; so, no one should die even in 34 days from a lack of food.*

Question: How do you come off your fast?

Answer: *Very good question...and, a most important one. Most professionals who supervise fasts agree that one should come off a fast on liquids. My recommendation is borrowed from Alvenia Fulton, N.D. ("The Queen-Mother of the Wholistic Movement"), who supervised Dick Gregory's early fasts. She encourages drinking one quart of fresh (organic) grape juice immediately after ending the fast. By contrast, Dr. Vetrano is more comfortable with vegetable juice, as more "sugar causes gas and pain" in some people. One should take only liquids one day for every three days he or she fasted.*

Question: How do you deal with hunger?

Answer: *What you call 'hunger' is really "withdrawal symptoms" from the addictive substances in the foods you consume. Once your body has been cleansed, you will experience an entirely different type of 'hunger.' If you are* *fasting for the first time, or even on a repeat fast, the sensation ("desire for food") should end by mid-day, certainly by the second day of fasting. After that, you will not feel "a sense of hunger."*

Question: Is fasting a dangerous thing to do?

Answer: *Not any more than sleeping is dangerous. We all fast when we sleep, when we are sick, when we are praying, during lent and at other times. There seems to be no special 'dangers' that might be attributed to fasting. However, persons who are insulin diabetics or are otherwise long term consumers of other drugs or chemicals might experience some adverse effects from those substances, especially when the 'cover' of food is taken away. For this reason any such person should seek professional guidance prior to attempting any prolonged fasting.*

Question: How do I start back eating?

Answer: *This question should be viewed in connection with my answer to the question of "ending the fast." First food should be fruit juice, vegetable juice or light soup. Next food should be raw fruit, perhaps some vegetables or sprouts; and so-called "solid foods" should not be resumed until after the liquid feeding days have passed, and at least one "all-fruit day."*

Question: Does your stomach shrink?

Answer: *The body is 'dynamic' (ever changing), so it is reasonable that going without contents for a time, the stomach will contract somewhat. However, what is more important for you to understand is that when you change what you eat, and chew your food properly, you will require less food for satisfaction than what you needed before your fast. You come to the point where you eat until you are satisfied, rather than until you are "full."*

Question: If I become 'light headed,' what should I do?

Answer: *The same thing you would do, whether you were fasting or not. Generally, you would want to cut your activities to allow the 'light headedness' to subside. If you are fasting when it happens, you might take a 10 to 15 minute rest. Also you might take a drink of water, swishing it about in the mouth* *before swallowing. By all means remain calm, focus on your overall feelings and concentrate on relaxing your mind and your body.*

Question: Can anyone supervise a fast?

Answer: *While fasting is a God-given right, and an essential medium in the healing process (animals on the great plains, or in the forests, do it routinely), our society is so filled with laws, and interest groups, and people pulling after our "consumer dollars," different factions espouse "Red Flag Alarms," most of which have little to do with you or your well being. But, because of these "cautions," it is advisable to consult a professional if you intend fasting for longer than 3 or 4 days.*

Question: How do you know how long to fast?

Answer: *The length of one's fast should focus on two considerations: 1) How much experience you have fasting and 2) What is your objective for fasting. If you are 'cleansing,' a minimum of three days on pure water (distilled) only should be a good start. If you are attempting to recover from a cold or flu or some other symptoms, you might fast until the symptoms are gone. This could be 4, 5, 7, 11, 15, 19, 23 or even more days. My longest fast was 30 days on water only; and that time I was just 'cleansing.'*

Question: Can children fast with safety?

Answer: *Age or sex has little to do with fasting. However, children sometimes consume things adults don't know about. Since fasting is natural to all human beings, any violent or adverse reaction during a fast suggests you look elsewhere for the cause. A child will often fast a day or more on his or her own, even without adults knowing about it. Some go for longer periods, sometimes evoking what is often referred to as "anorexia."*

Question: Is fasting a medical procedure?

Answer: *No, I don't see that it is. "Medical procedures, treatments or practices" must have one or more of the following elements: 1) Prescription of drugs or pharmaceuticals or* *'medications;' 2) Examinations and calibrations, tests and measurements (to predetermined norms); or 3) The surgical modification and/or removal of part or all of a portion of the body, or the repair or mending of some body part or function. Now, this is a layman's definition; but it is enough to exclude fasting from being classified as "a medical procedure."*

Question: Is suggesting to someone what he or she might do about a certain physical or mental problem considered 'practicing medicine?'

Answer: *I am not sure how your question is related to fasting, but it seems to me the answer to that type of question is not unrelated to how biblical 'interpretations' are made. It depends upon the person, motivation and purposes to be served. As with the Bible, one can 'prove' just about any argument about just about anything. If properly motivated, certain persons probably could 'prove' that grandmother Reatter was "practicing medicine" when she 'prescribed' chicken soup and rest when we children had colds.*

Question: How often would you recommend fasting?

Answer: *This would depend, as all things should, upon what is your purpose or motivation for fasting in the first place. If you are changing the way you eat, drink, exercise, and rest, I would suggest 3- and 4-day fasting, once a month as convenient. For assisting or not interfering with maximum cleansing by the organism, one should try to create as restful, supportive, warm and clean an environment as available, then fast for as long as is consistent with fasting experience and knowledge about fasting. For me, I try to do at least one 9-to-15-day fast every six months.*

Question: Is it a good idea to have someone else to fast with?

Answer: *It is a good idea to learn all you can about fasting; to be clear about your objectives; to verify your information; and, of course, to share with kindred spirits this joyful thing you will be doing from time to time.*

Question: Let's say that I need help during my fast, who do I call?

Answer: *If you intend to fast longer than over night or a day or two, I suggest you read books on fasting so you will be as informed as possible. If you do not have time to inform yourself, perhaps you should forego fasting completely. On the other hand, if you have questions before you commence a fast, you can call a number of professional associations and/or individuals. The Rest of Your Life Health Retreat, PO Box 102, Barksdale, TX (where Dr. Vetrano is located) is my most highly recommended facility. But, there are others found in the literature and on the Internet.*

Fasting Overview

The 'common sense' definition of *fasting* is "the abstinence of food and substance, or a reduction in normal consumption." This goes on around the clock, for 24-hour periods. A dictionary definition is "to keep from eating all or certain foods; to eat very little or nothing." Either definition lends itself to the variety of practices known, generally, as healing fasts (as in the animal kingdom), religious fasts (as with spiritual activities), fruit fasts, juice fasts, wheat grass fasts, brown rice fasts, soup and crackers fasts and, of course, water-only fasts.

Reasons for fasting are as varied as the types of fasts: to lose weight, to grow spiritually, to enhance prayer, to cleanse the body, to purge the mind, to heal the body or to recover from some debilitating state.

Hygienic ***fasting*** proposes a technique to be used primarily as a 'preventive' lifestyle practice which, when extended, is—in the view of Natural Hygiene—the most effective method of overcoming acute, chronic and even degenerative disease conditions.

John H. Tilden, MD, the son of a physician, received his medical education at the Eclectic Medical Institute, Cincinnati, Ohio, a medical school founded in 1830 as a protest against the allopathic and homeopathic schools of medicine of that time. He has described disease conditions as various "stages of toxemia." Dr. Tilden asks the question we ascribe to hygienic fasting:

"What more can be asked of a health care system than that it simplifies the cause of disease, making it understandable to all open-minded lay minds?"

Misconceptions can help lead to the onset of disease conditions. The notion that one has to 'eat to live' leads to overeating, a deadly practice at its worst. The consumption of 'legal drugs' like aspirin, salt, alcohol, caffeine, 'sweeteners' and chemical-laden flesh foods makes 98% of Americans unhealthy, despite their abundant eating.

A growing number of credible researchers and scientists is more and more identifying so-called "HIV-AIDS" as nothing more than "a description of a body dying" from the over consumption of prescription and other drugs (and chemicals).

In 1974, T. C. Fry wrote, "54% of all Americans die of heart disease...autopsies of our most fit young men who died on the Korean battlefields showed that 77% of them already had heart disease. About one billion visits are made to physicians annually, and about 4,500,000 people each year are poisoned so seriously by their physicians as to require hospitalization!"

A lot of these 'dismal statistics' are already widely known. What people with melanin seem less willing to accept is that sugar is not their friend; bread is not a good food for humans; all types of drugs poison the organism; non-organically produced and cooked foods are injurious to health; and, finally, "over 3,000,000,000 (that's three billion) sleeping pills are consumed annually. An estimated 13,000,000,000 (13 billion) barbiturate and amphetamine pills are ingested annually (as of 1974!). Is anyone out there really interested in what is killing people with melanin? Or, is the 'hypnotic spell' of the "death with dignity" movement too pervasive to surface from beneath tons of public deception? Drugs and chemicals are killing more Americans, for example, than "foreign enemies" or atomic weapons ever will!

This chapter has been proclaimed as "a God-send" to many who have been long-term substance abusers, and those attempting to overcome military, workplace or other forms of toxicity. And, while we in Natural Hygiene know that hygienic fasting (as a periodic supplement to a wellness lifestyle) prevents acute disease and ameliorates chronic disease conditions, fasting—when begun in time, and is continued long enough—offers real hope of surviving degenerative disease conditions as well.

Each individual, considering his or her options, must stop at nothing to become as informed as possible. In the final analysis, each individual must assume responsibility for what happens to his or her life. If the present trends continue, individual "freedom of treatment modalities" will be corroded to "only conventional options;" and in a society where allopathic and homeopathic practitioners are less and less "subject to legal redress for malpractice," and where the pharmaceutical and chemical industries get away "Scot free," Mother God will surely only help those who help themselves.

'Big Brother' is a part of the system. Educating oneself about ***the nature and purpose of disease*** and how to prevent disease, or how to resolve disease, is surely the best 'insurance' one can buy. That this chapter will save fortunes is desirable; that it will save lives is the real 'miracle!'

Introducing H.A.R.A.

Dr. Herbert M. Shelton, the "father of natural hygiene," held that "all diseases are the same disease" and that "healing is an innate body process." What Dr. Shelton advocates is educating individuals so that they may *assist* the body in recovering when it shows signs of 'toxic overload.' This philosophy is at the heart of the author's own Organic Wellness Crusade educational methodology.

Hurdle-Antechachexy Regenerative Agent (H.A.R.A.) is the only recommended "aid" to enhance organic cleansing. The tonic grown and marketed by the Organic Wellness Crusade (PO Box 7219, Beverly Hills, CA 90212-7219), as an inducement for hygienic fasting, especially by those who are used to "taking something" or "doing something" as a part of the 'therapy process.' H.A.R.A is distributed exclusively by the **Reatter**

Lonon Family Trust of Sylvania, Georgia (***Distributor*, Ms. Flora Jenkins**, ***1507 Dell Street, Savannah, GA 31401, Tel. 912-233-6964).*** As has been said, the tonic enhances the body's own "life force." Recognizing that individuals are 'creatures of habit,' a "sweet aloe juice" concentrate is obtained, from which the tonic is made that stimulates the body's own healing process; and when drunk while employing our organic wellness fasting technique, various positive results are sure to come into evidence.

In treating his sports injuries clients at International Academy of Sportscience in Gennep, The Netherlands, Prof. Bert van Wingerden says, "We often find it necessary to, first, put the patient or client on a 'detoxification' fast of water only, to clear the system of medications—pain killers, antibiotics, stimulants, barbiturates, steroids, stabilizers—for as long as three weeks." He continued, "Using this procedure, coupled with the use of certain electro-medical devices (electronic machines that reduce pain and enhance healing), we achieve results that have received acclaim from around the world."

A Word of Caution

Even though 'fasting' is something done by every living creature (during sleep, during sickness, during abstinence from food and/or drink, during religious celebrations, during sex), *hygienic or organic wellness fasting may not be for everyone.* You should check your intentions with your personal advisor. Where many days fasting is contemplated, seek professional guidance from a student of natural hygiene. Dr. Vetrano worked very closely with Dr. Herbert M. Shelton for some 15 years; she is available for professional guidance (P.O. Box 102, Barksdale, TX 78828).

Persons who are highly toxic, those who have been or who are addicted to chemical or other substances, and those consuming medications or herbs or drugs of any kind should be as informed as possible. We recommend reading *Helping Hand: A Guide to Healthy Living* (Anderson, 1992), *Fasting Can Save*

Your Life (Shelton, H. M.), *Toxemia: The Basic Cause of Disease* (Tilden, John H.) for starters.

When employing the Organic Wellness Crusade's fasting technique for the first time, it is advisable not to fast longer than three days. After that, judging from your results, you may repeat the technique, even extending the period of time to 5, 7, 9, 11 or more days with experienced and professional guidance. However, in the early stages of hygienic fasting advise someone close of your intentions, activities and progress. And, remember, longer fasts might be accompanied by a 15-minute daily Seitz bath.

Preparation for Hygienic Fasting

Prepare your body for fasting, just as you would prepare for swimming. You don't just "jump right into the water" in your street clothes. You decide you are going to go get into the water (and swim, maybe!). Next, you plan when you are going; you dress yourself for "being in the water," and you make other supportive arrangements you feel necessary to maximize your time "in the water." By so doing, you already start mental and physical relaxation, lowering your energy generation to a calmer level. Now, after all of this you are ready to get yourself to the water's edge, and stick your toe in to test the temperature!

In organic wellness or hygienic fasting, so too must we prepare our minds and our space for the important decision we are in the process of making. Finally, when everything is ready—all paraphernalia and our 'mental swimsuit' is on—we "stick in our toe, to test the temperature!"

Three or four days before the fast is to begin, cut back on 'normal consumption' of food, drink or other substances. One or two days before the healing fast begins, consume only liquid foods—organic (or, at least, fresh squeezed!) fruit or vegetable juices, but no blended nuts or other solid foods; and absolutely no herbs or drugs (unless, of course, you are under care of a licensed professional, treating you, by your consent, in the manner he or she has been trained and is, therefore, licensed).

Organic wellness or hygienic fasting is not recommended for persons who 'are standing in dire need,' especially those who are "standing at death's door." When you go swimming in the face of a hurricane you are truly in a desperate situation. We feel for them, but dare not give them 'false hope.' The organic wellness or hygienic fasting technique works best to *prevent* such desperation. Once the body's condition is visibly deteriorating, 'Cause and Effect,' the Supreme Law of the Universe, comes into play. Not even Mother God 'can stop' the course of preordained Time.

In other words, if the hurricane is on the scene already, and one's time cycle is visibly concluding, to swim or not to swim is almost academic! We say 'almost' because in Natural Hygiene, we believe—as we do well know—so long as the dynamic human organism is alive and functioning independently—at whatever level of efficiency—there is some benefit to be derived. Perhaps, however, this benefit comes not from deliberate fasting, but from "two actions" which aid healing: 1) stopping the poisoning, and 2) eliminating retained toxins.

Dynamics of Fasting

First, *stopping the consumption* of that which poisons or leads to the poisoning of the organism, and second, *resting the organism*—mind and body—minimizing disruptions and interference: this is *how we assist* the organism in its own healing activities. Therefore, the first part of your preparation should be equipping yourself with reliable information. You need to know what has been said (written) up to now; and you need to know much, much more; but immediately, you need to know that when the healing activity is taking place, the organism will begin casting off or eliminating unwanted 'stuff,' so-called "toxins," through and from its organs (skin, lungs, kidneys, liver, intestine, bladder, eyes, tongue, genitals, and the blood, our largest and most vital body organ!).

The dumping of this 'stored garbage' takes different forms in different individuals. One might experience pimples on the skin and face, or even boils; still others might notice blurred vision, or foul smelling genitals or feet; and for nearly all, the fecal elimination will slow or stop. It is important to be informed and advised so that when these "strange things" start happening to you, they do not cause undue alarm and, therefore, will not disrupt *your psychic rhythm*, permitting your organism to continue its cleansing, with minimum interference from you.

An annotated bibliography of recommended source material is included at the end of this volume. Remember, as the poet has said, "A little learning is a dangerous thing; so drink deeply from the fountain of" information.

Beginning the Organic Wellness Fast

When you are prepared for your fast—and you have NOT attempted to "flush" your organic colon as one would flush an inorganic commode! —you are about to commence one of the most important, and most life giving experiences you'll ever have! By drinking only H.A.R.A./tm (**Hurdle Antechechexy Regenerative Agent**) and purified water, while abstaining from all other substances, you have made "an agreement" with your organism that "I will not, nor will I permit anyone else to interfere!"

And your contract is not complete until you can let go of mental disturbances: *fear of dying* (from not eating food!); *tormenting notions* out of the subconscious mind concerning a wide variety of "negative effects;" *confusion* caused by herbalists, healers, friends, old folks—even physicians who mean well, and those who feel 'threatened' by your independent action! Do not be alarmed or surprised as these *anxieties* appear in your consciousness. Be steadfast and they will quickly disappear. And the morning and the evening of your first day's organic wellness fast would have been behind you.

By the second day, your 'lightheadedness' should subside or disappear (if, in fact, you experience such phenomenon). Your body might want a 10 to 15 minute rest in mid-afternoon. By now you will have nearly lost any sense of "hunger." As your body prepares itself to begin cleansing, it waits to 'verify' your commitment to cooperate. By the end of the second day, your body will know whether you are 'serious,' and if you are cleansing activities will begin to become evident.

Evidence of this cleansing activity should be of little concern to those using this fasting technique for the first time. It is to be expected if urine becomes a darker color; normal fecal elimination may not occur; the body will begin to feel lighter and more 'energetic.' For many, breath will become foul. At this time natural peppermint, chlorophyll, sesame, anise, parsley or other organic aids can make life more pleasant for those around you! A liquid chlorophyll drop is recommended as an overall "breath aid."

Colleagues, friends and family may not understand what you are doing, or why you are doing this, or what is supposed to happen while you do what you do. They often show their own anxieties, even more so because they feel so ill equipped to either understand or provide expertise. You will have to hear them out; just know they are speaking from what they feel is genuine concern. Tell them *what they need to know* (you are following a 'proven technique' and professional assistance is just a phone call away). They need to know, too, your personal commitment to and understanding of what you are doing.

After you have reached your *3-day minimum commitment*, do each additional day without commitment—one day at a time. Finally, decide the day before if you can, that "Tomorrow, I will end this cleansing fasting." This will send a signal to your brain to tell all body processes they have 24 hours to begin gearing up for a resumption of regular functions.

And, because your organic factory ("machine and equipment") has been 'idle' for some time, you do not want to go at "full speed" right away. This is why you will come off or *end your organic wellness fast by drinking only liquids* (one full day of liquids for every three days you abstained from 'normal' foods).

During Your Cleansing Fast

When a proper cleansing fast is conducted, many wonderful results have been reported, time and again, over the years, by many different supervisors of fasts, practitioners and professionals. Yours should be no different.

It is important, however, that you are properly prepared to go on an extended fast, even for just three days! If you have been heavily on medications, controlled substances or other concentrated intake, of whatever nature, it will be even more important for you to have 'prepared' your body as many days in advance of commencing the fasting as possible.

Nor is there much difference in preparing the body mentally. If you have been long under 'stress,' have been depressed or "kind of low" for a long time, it will be important to spend some advance time building up your spirit, feeling better about yourself and what wonderful thing you are about to do for yourself!

One of the most obvious results during the fasting is that you <u>can</u> expect to lose weight. Persons who "are retaining a lot of water" can lose 10 pounds or more in one day. When I played sports in college, for example, on a single 'football Saturday,' I've lost as much as 12 pounds! Of course, some kids lost more, some less. I was not only 'fasting' but engaged in strenuous physical activity as well. Nonetheless, the first thing lost is the water; therefore, more of what 'water weight' comes off in the initial days of a longer fast. As the organism settles into its cleansing activities weight loss will average three-quarters of a pound per day (15 pounds lost in 20 days of fasting, for a person down to around 10% body fat, as I tend to be). Most Americans are far above 10% in body fat and will, therefore, tend to lose more poundage per day.

On the cleansing side of the ledger, many so-called and popularly identified "diseases" will disappear during fasting, depending upon the individual and, of course, other variables (some knowable, some not knowable). Depending on which professional you ask, or what reference book you read, or upon who is speaking, it is not unusual to hear some of the following **"healing probabilities:"**

In 3 to 4 days of hygienic fasting, the organism is able to sufficiently 'dump unwanted stuff' such that "the symptoms" may no longer be visible for elimination activities referred to as common cold, vaginal-uterine infections, hot flashes, inflammation of the reproductive organs, painful urination, lemon-sized tumors, many skin ailments, pimples and acne, PMS, uncomfortable menses, minor pancreas irritation, headache, fatigue, allergies, strep throat, mucous accumulation, colitis, Psoriasis, Eczema, dry and scaly skin, hyperglycemia, water retention, clogged liver-spleen-pancreas, gout, Edema, urinary infection, arthritis, excess toxicity, vaginal yeast infection, excessive bleeding, hemorrhoids, slow nose bleeds, inflamed ulcers, diarrhea, irregular blood pressure, and increased strength of "the immune system."

Hygienic **fasting for 5 to 7 days** has been credited with partial relief from discomfort and pain of arthritis, rheumatism or bursitis, arteriosclerosis, acidosis due to accumulation of toxins, flu, exhaustion, depression, gastric discomfort, fever, palpitation of the heart, coronary heart disease, congestive heart disease, arteriosclerosis, angina, Parkinson's disease, myocardial infraction, hypertension, emotional stress and anxiety, acute nervousness, erysipelas, hives, shingles, twitching, tic syndrome, migraine headache, acute pain, acute toxicity, tetanus, venereal disease, moles, viral warts, body odor and halitosis, sore throat, varicose veins, bowel congestion, jaundice, hepatitis, cirrhosis, sluggish spleen-pancreas-gall bladder, intestinal spasms, and adds even more strength to the "immune system."

Seven to 11 days of organic wellness fasting is said to have an impact on physical weakness, lack of stamina, sterility, poor memory, hypoglycemia, prostate problems, enlarged prostate, inflammation of the prostate, pain in the lower extremities, parasitic infection, insomnia, weight loss, high cholesterol, swollen joints, upset stomach, heartburn, duodenal-peptic-gastric ulcers, poor digestion or circulation, congestion, constipation, eye and vision discomfort, early formation cataracts, glaucoma, sore, and greater strengthening of 'the immune system."

The Seitz Bath

During fasts that last longer than three days, the daily Seitz bath helps get rid of material gathered in the large intestine or colon. However, care should be taken. So important is managing the Seitz bath, we pause here to describe *the organic wellness method.* Fill the bathtub (while sitting) to waist height with hot water (100-102 degrees). Remain sitting for some 15 to 20 minutes. Get out of the tub slowly, allowing the water to drain from the tub. Dry yourself, and rest or "cool down" five to ten minutes (until you are no longer perspiring). Keep yourself warm and comfortable, and covered.

At the time of the daily Seitz bath, during your fasting, or even during normal times, it is important to know you should not "push down" when passing fecal matter. The helpful way is to *draw in the stomach muscles.* In this manner, you best assist the body in smoothly 'pushing forth' excremental matter into the anal passage way and out into the commode. One danger of "pushing down" is that it is a primary contributor to tissue lesions, which are referred to as "hemorrhoids."

Results of Longer Fasting Periods

If you have used the OWC fasting method before, or any system that worked for you, and you consider yourself 'an experienced faster,' **over a period of 12 to 15 days** on pure water and/or H.A.R.A./tm, there can be significant relief from the effects of general poisoning, radiation, microwave exposure, heavy metal toxicity, air pollution, water pollution, processed foods, "fast foods," chemicals and drugs, alcohol, caffeine, salt and pepper, tobacco products, dairy products, animal products, home and workplace pollutants, gallstones, severe constipation, appendicitis, isocheim heart disease, thyroid malfunction, hypothalamus, adrenal-pineal-pituitary-lymph glands sluggishness, and the organism's relative inability to throw off toxins improves.

During 16 to 21 days, some point to tremendous improvement in their rheumatoid arthritis, over-toxicity, emotional and work-related stress, exhaustion or "chronic stress/fatigue syndrome," and noticeable improvement in their mental alertness and overall body function.

Twenty-two to 25 days and many wonderful things seem to occur: greater self-esteem, increased motivation, higher energy level, better memory, sharper mind, less sign of senility, clearer skin and a great overall sense of well being! Even longer fasting has been credited with regulating cholesterol, reducing discomfort from asthma-hay fever-sinus, reducing noticeable food and chemical allergies, aiding dislocations-atrophied muscles-disc deteriorations, and tightening up loose flesh.

While there are some reasonable claims of overcoming cancer, A.I.D.S., diabetes, stroke, high blood pressure, leukemia, multiple sclerosis, impotency and sterility, and other so-called "chronic" and "degenerative" disease conditions through hygienic fasting, one must do individual research and experimentation—always holding to the "rule of common sense." This is how one really learns what is true, with the guidance of a doctor of Natural Hygiene.

Those who wish personal testimonies may contact organizations such as the Organic Wellness Crusade (http://www.organicwellness.com and www.healthfullivingintl.org) or local "holistic" organizations which support and subscribe to the scientific proof that the human organism has within itself its own "life force" for healing itself, to the extent humans do not interfere.

Ending Your Fast

How you end your fast is critical. You do not want to shock your system. You want to allow time for readjustment. Those of you who have worked in factories which shut down for a time, or those involved in education know how it is the first day or so after a shut down or school vacation period ends!

As part of your preparation for this fast, you located a quick source of organic grape or other berry juice. The berry juice that you secure should be unfiltered (if not organic) and you should clearly see the solid pulp of the berries floating in or settled at the bottom of the glass container. You might even dilute the fruit juice with an equal amount of distilled water. It some instances, it is preferable to use fresh vegetable juice, or even vegetable broth.

You will EAT (chew and swallow, slowly—not gulp!) this pint (16oz) of grape juice until it is gone. For the rest of the day, continue to drink fruit or vegetable juices; then continue "eating' berry juice, fruit juice, vegetable juice, one day for every three days you fasted. If you fasted only three days, the 4th day you will Eat berry juice mainly. If you fasted 5 days, you will Eat liquids for 2 additional days. You may switch to other fruit or vegetable juices on the second day, if you prefer.

If you fasted 8 or 9 days, you may eat berry juice to end the fast, other fruit or vegetable juice the second day after the ending of the fast, or warm or cold broth or very light soup the third day after your fast ended.

On the first day of "solid food," let it be organic or fresh FRUITS in season. **Always try to eat *one type* of fruit (or vegetable per feeding)**; but feed as many times as you would like. Take note, your body will NOT want the quantity of food you consumed prior to beginning your fast! Eat melons first and bananas last. And, until you have resumed your 'normal' eating routine, avoid dried, concentrated and "sunfired" fruits, because the concentrated natural sugars should come only when you've been eating "regularly" for some time.

A further word about "ending your fast." Do not be surprised if you do not end your fast when you first say you will. Very often, when you come more into harmony with your organism, decisions about what to do or what not to do are no longer made "in your head." *Your organism takes over and dictates what will be!* And, you learn to listen and to respect "your body's decisions." So, prepare yourself for the emergence of a 'new force' within. This is the *life force, which* is submerged in all of us. Organic wellness or therapeutic fasting is a way of freeing up this force. You'll know when it is happening!

After Ending Your Cleansing Fast

Do not be surprised if you find yourself not wanting to eat certain foods. Certainly, your "life force" will tell you very clearly: "I do not want 'this' or 'that' inside of me!" It will speak like a determined woman; make no mistake about it! No one will need to interpret anything for you. And each time you do another fast, of equal time or longer, your "life force" will appear even stronger.

Your stomach will seem smaller. You will not want to eat as much as you did before. You will realize how much time is "wasted" during the feeding ritual. You will find the more you CHEW the less you will want to eat, and the more you will notice the benefits of eating less. You come to feel invincible! <u>You gain control over your life</u>. Soon, you will be able to float through life—unaffected by the "diseases" of humankind, and tuned into a higher spiritual domain in which you, alone, reside in the company of your own loving and protective ("HARA") *Life Force*!

Remember, we are here for each other. Identify a contact person to call if you want support, have questions, or need clarification. Call *before*, not after your uncertainty. If you want to tell of your joy, or if you just want to share financial resources in support of the Organic Wellness Crusade, you may write to P.O. Box 7219, Beverly Hills, CA 90212-7219 or email to <u>truth@organicwellness.com</u>.

I will end on a rhetorical, hypothetical note: As I sit listening to the frying "sizzle" of hot grease (animal or vegetable oils), my 'other ear' hears the screaming siren of an emergency vehicle! (Time lapse to the future, when "heart attack" occurs).

If knowing what leads to future distress is unimportant, then why not end the pretense? Why continue to financially support—and in the best form and style, I might add—an army of "prostitutes" who are called "health care professionals," who seem to know, also, that prescribing and treating is a kind of "game," a highly profitable ritual.

This 'ritual' brings together "those who know what causes their troubles, but show little interest in prevention" with those "who rally to diagnose, prescribe and treat," with little reliance upon any 'cure.'

Chapter Eighteen

Anderson Postulates

One, no matter how well we live...or how poorly, we will not "get out of this rat race alive." So, our nobler objective is to experience optimum wellness and happiness while we are here.

Two, we cannot experience optimum wellness so long as we persist in poisoning ourselves (or permitting others to poison us!).

Three, the 'wellness issue' is not, and never was about *how long* we might live; it is, rather, about the *quality* of our lives while we live.

Four, once poisoned (as we all have been since infancy!), our wellness salvation lies in an effective routine of on-going, systemic detoxification, which includes, of course, adequate exercise and regular elimination.

Five, shortly into a managed wellness consciousness, and deliberate action plan, we receive such benefits from which no one is ever able to separate us again.

Six, the formula is simple: we stop the poisoning, become conscious of eliminating already stored toxins, and develop a lifestyle that makes detoxification as routine as daily cleanliness.

Seven, the world is being led to believe that a seldom-present "virus" called 'HIV' is the *cause* of AIDS. This is a deliberate deception, according to Prof. Duesberg, T.C. Fry, and others.

Eight, such belief, therefore, is dulling public sensitivity to increasing "mass murder-by-default," and there is little or no public outrage!

Nine, "What If...?" deaths from so-called AIDS are really the consequences of consuming drugs (medications, inoculations, vaccinations, 'recreational drugs,' traditional pharmaceuticals and prescriptions), and chemical poisoning (internal from a denatured diet, malnutrition, starvation, protein poisoning, polluted drinking water, war and industrial chemicals ingested) and externally from environmental and atmospheric poisoning (vehicular exhaust, factory pollution, air conditioning systems, toxic wastes, micro-waves, loud noises, natural gases and combinations of the above)? Question is: can you ignore the impact of all of the above, in favor of the questionable existence of a causal "virus?" Remember, Duesberg and others have proven "'HIV' causes nothing" (except: panic, distortion, deception, mental devastation, and a financial whirlwind!).

Ten, if the above is true—*and there is scientific proof available*—"permitting" the deaths of tens of thousands is an act of "murder-by-default," a form of genocide!

Eleven, this killing campaign is disguised in the cloak of the Hitlerian Big Lie: "HIV, the virus that causes AIDS!"

Twelve, God help a world that cannot seem to learn what Adolph Hitler taught: *"If you want people to believe a lie, tell it over and over and over!"*

Thirteen, "*Just say no to drugs*" commits the lie of omission, leading the public to believe—falsely—in a 'resolve' which is **the world's largest free advertising campaign** for a product—drugs! No thanks to the "Just say no to drugs" ads, children everywhere *either know about drugs*, or they are made curious! The rest of the story is reflected in public health and death statistics.

Fourteen, drug consumption is too profitable and too close to big commercial interests and big government to reasonably expect *law enforcement* to 'protect' generations of future addicts.

Fifteen, therefore, a multi-trillion dollar industry has been created, and every so-called AIDS death is placed squarely at the feet of the drug/pharmaceutical/chemical cartel and their political cohorts.

Sixteen, the largest pro-drug advertisement in the world is free: "Just say no to drugs!" Everyone of us who 'promotes' that message is a co-conspirator in the scheme to "poison, disenfranchise, and profit from the demise" of millions.

Seventeen, by resolving the issues raised in these postulates, peoples of the world—*those with obvious melanin*—approach regaining control over their health, wellness, longevity and, consequently, significantly preventing the occurrence of disease conditions in their lives, and in their countries.

Author's Equations

As a high school student, geometry was one of my favorite subjects. In fact, it became monumental when a teacher revealed a promise he had made to earlier classes: "When one of my students solves a geometry problem in fewer steps than I do, I will resign my position and move on!" Until that quiet, unsuspecting day, I was one student who "enjoyed geometry."

The class was reviewing problems from the day's homework assignment. Our teacher called a few of us to the chalk board because he wanted to review one problem before the entire class. He made a point to call me up to the board, among other students. He announced to the class that a problem he solved in twelve steps, I had solved in eight; and, he was certain my solution was in error.

After several attempts to "prove" errors in the development of my problem, our teacher turned to those of us gathered at the chalk board and declared: "The problem is correct; Anderson did it in eight steps. I made a promise years ago that whenever one of my students did this to me, I would resign. That time has come...." With those surprising remarks, my teacher walked out of the classroom, down to the office where he resigned, and was never seen at Benjamin Franklin High School in Philadelphia again. I graduated and went on to college on full scholarship.

It was sometime before I became really aware of what had happened. It was finally explained to me by my Guidance Counselor, Mrs. Payton. I understood and soon put the entire matter into perspective. What rang true, even more so, was that what we called 'corollaries,' or in Logic "premises" were still true. "*Things equal to the same thing are equal to each other*," is one I remember very clearly. In Logic, "An argument which is based on a false premise will remain false," is a paraphrase of a 'truism.' In Natural Hygiene, according to T. C. Fry, "Disease does not occur unless it is caused." And, for this writer, *where the causes remain constant, so too will the effects continue consistent.*

Un-eliminated poisons in the food chain lead to cancer; drugs consumed and retained lead to the defenseless condition known as "full blown AIDS."

The following are believed by me to be just as fundamental, just as sound as a corollary or a premise. I believe that the following are true equations:

HIV/AIDS = Accumulated drugs/chemicals; poisoning in the lymphatic system.

Cancer/s = Poisoning from dietary factors and mental stress, largely.

Cancer in Children = Poisoning from S.A.D. (Standard American Diet) and deficiencies received from parent (male) and/or from parents (male and female).

Cardiovascular = Heart vessels (arteries) damage from animal fats, caffeine, nicotine, alcohol and other drugs.

Heart Disease = Atrophy from sedentary and stressful lifestyle, including animal-based dietary consumptions.

Diabetes = Insulin reduction or depletion from dietary and/or emotional stress.

High Blood Pressure = Clogged arteries, primarily from accumulated animal fats.

MS = Poisoning from deposits of metals and/or metallic chemicals and drugs.

Hypertension = Systemic responses to accumulated animal by-products and internally produced body chemicals.

Poisoning = Effects from substances un-used and un-eliminated by the organism. Anything consumed without nutrient or utilization potential.

Virus = "Dead" organic matter, the 'scale' or 'crust' ("dead skin") of cells that die daily (but are replenished by the organism). Latin, "poison;" substance without life.

Migraine = Blood vessel blockage to the brain (to stop or slow the flow of poisons already in the blood stream).

Contagion = Magic or "Hocus Pocus!" The "illusion" upon which the medical establishment depends for its perceived survival; a false construct that absolves the 'guilty' of responsibility.

Birth Defects = Parental (male) drugs/chemicals "transgressions" (as in 'professional athletes,' military personnel, factory workers, and sometimes mothers who frequently consume 'medications').

Anxiety = Chemical imbalance resulting from "toxic overload."

Neuroses = Stress responses to accumulated "mental garbage."

Psychoses = Results produced by deranged mental faculties (from trauma or systemic malfunction) the results of 'psychic stuff' not eliminated from the psychic system.

Symptoms = Evidences of a toxic state. 'Suppressing one symptom leads to another, even more critical than was the former (and perhaps 'hidden' from view for quite some time).

Alzheimers = Death of brain cells, resulting from the accumulated effects of ingesting simple sugars (as in desserts), and metals (aluminum, lead, bio-carbons, drugs or medications), and sometimes from head injuries.

Kidney Disease = Functional shutdown, from accumulated effects of Scotch whiskey, alcohol and chemical compounds.

Cholesterol = Clotting grease (animal fat) in the arteries, which is the substance of animal products (the only source of the so-called "bad cholesterol").

Stroke = Oxygen-deprived crisis in the brain, usually brought on by cholesterol-laden blood vessels, particularly at a stressful time.

Impotency = Excess mental and physical "baggage," hindering normal organic functioning.

Sterility = Deranged systemic structures due to accumulated toxicity (sometimes due to structural damage, from medical procedure/s or other traumatic interference).

Fibroids = Accumulated tissue, which has not been discarded due to constant dietary, emotional and mental stress.

Chronic Fatigue Syndrome = Enervation (over expenditure of nerve energy) affecting specific, observed and/or non-specific body/mind functions. The "condition" described as "physical/mental exhaustion."

Disease = Manifestation of poisoning, its specific and varied 'symptoms, diagnoses and unique processes'—all such cases having a common cause, **poisoning**, and a common remedy, **detoxification** (except for degenerative conditions).

Chronic Disease = Reoccurring symptoms resulting from toxic overload.

Acute Disease = An initiated "process" that, unless slowed, will lead to the earlier demise of the organism.

Degenerative Disease = Compromised status of body or mind function that signifies (more or less) permanent damage at the structural or cellular level.

Starvation = Prolonged deprivation of nutritious food.

Malnutrition = Under-nourishment resulting from insufficient nutrients in foods consumed.

Protein Poisoning = The deadliest form of organic poisoning, generally from over consumption of animal protein (at all levels).

Crisis = Imminent threat to organic balance.

Latent = Lying in wait.

Dormant = Evident inactivity.

Direct = Straight forward.

Indirect = Roundabout.

Organic = Totally natural.

Inorganic = Non-living matter.

Voluntary = Stimulated.

Involuntary = Not stimulated.

Manifestation = Observable, visible evidence.

Senile = Incapacity from accumulated effects.

Death/Dying = Transition of organic matter.

Prognosis = Speculation of future condition.

Healthfulness/Wellness = Slowest possible systemic poisoning.

Shock = Sudden impact.

Environmental Factors = Communal phenomena adversely affecting health and well being, thereby contributing to the build-up of toxic overload.

Pollution = Poison sub-systems able to negatively impact the world of living things, especially of humans (for our purposes).

Skin Cancer = Acute ulceration on most vulnerable skin, from irritation, radiation and/or chemical stress.

AIDS Epidemic = Possibly a military tactic to 'neutralize' and control populations (people of the world who are readily identified by the presence of melanin in their skin).

Irradiation = The application of low levels of nuclear by-products on food stuffs, ostensibly to preserve shelf life, but actually is a slow killer of white blood cells, leading ultimately to the condition generally known as "full-blown AIDS."

Genetically Engineered Foods = Items designated as "foods" that have been altered, therefore "created" in a 'lab.' An 'altered food substance' that is substantially poisonous when consumed by humans.

Author's Postscript

Since you've gotten this far through the volume, and through your own life, I owe you the very best that I have in me. This parting stricture: What we refer to as "disease" is not an 'enemy' to either humans or to creatures; it is rather 'living' testimony—confirmation—that Universal Law is operative in our universe. For, as my late mentor, T.C. Fry, so eloquently put it: "Sickness and disease will not occur so long as we do not engage the causal behaviors."

Perhaps the most plausible approach is for me to speak, as if to myself—as if I suffered from these self-same "afflictions, symptoms and disease conditions."

Believing, as I do, that 'afflictions' result from either **body storage** (accumulation) mostly; **trauma** too often; and, from **natural imperfection** occasionally, my keenest interest would be in determining what I can first do to begin—immediately—to neutralize the content of my body/mind which sustains the adverse condition so that its effects might be reversed! In other words, I would want to "***begin the slow, but systematic process of detoxifying my body/mind***," allowing me to get well again.

Since I truly believe "all diseases are the same disease," and what rids the body/mind of one set of symptoms will, most likely, get rid of other sets of symptoms as well, I would:

1. Immediately forego cooked foods (if I had not already done so!).
2. Eat only fruits, vegetables, nuts and seeds (raw and organically grown, to the extent possible).
3. Drink only distilled or carbon-filtered water.
4. Abstain from food (do a long fast) for as many days as practical, beyond three (on water only), and under trained supervision (yourself or some other person).
5. Exercise sufficiently to enhance body/mind elimination and overall function.
6. Consume an abundance of fresh air and sunshine sufficient to clean the lungs and invigorate the body.

7. Continue to keep warm, in a friendly environment.

8. Produce positive thoughts; clear any negative thoughts; **forgive** and forget; and think well of myself and of others (despite anything).

9. Seek out and verify reliable information; and continue to implement those principles into my lifestyle.

10. Decide—again—that non-traditional, hygienic recommendations shall be followed, "for better or for worse."

11. Make and keep peace with The Creator, "Mother Nature;" and improve upon the quality of life in all possible aspects.

12. Rest, sleep and recreate often and adequately, with others and alone.

13. Share whenever I can what I believe to be the best system of well being available to anyone—Natural Hygiene.

14. In short, I would—I do believe—become an extremist in the wellness lifestyle, which forms the core of my Natural Hygiene belief structure. **I would, in a word, practice what I preach!**

15.

Yours as an emancipated Organic Wellness Crusader, I remain

—Henry L. N. Anderson, Fruitarian and Natural Hygienist
August 21, 2002
(Happy Birthday Margie!)

Bibliography

Selected Annotations

1. Afrika, Llaila O., *African Holistic Health*, Silver Spring, MD 20914: Sea Island Information Group, Adesegun, Johnson & Koram Publishers, 1989.

-Complete herb remedy guide, 'dis-ease' treatments, nutrition, diet, wholistic perspectives, Africa herb history, self diagnosis, charts, wholistic sex laws, herpes and AIDS treatments, cocaine detox and foods that kill. Introduction by Dick Gregory.

2. Afua, Queen, *Heal Thyself with Health and Longevity*: New York, Heal Thyself Center, 1991.

-Something for everyone, in the name of 'fasting.' Filled with various references and descriptions of 'fasting and healing processes.'

3. Anderson, Henry L. N., Ed.D., *African, Born in America*. Beverly Hills, CA 90212-7219: BLI Publishing, 1993.

-A sociopolitical autobiography, exploring the life-span realities of growing up under the domination of white people, particularly as experienced in America. A keenly perspective series of responses on issues reflecting answers to the question: "What have I become (What can I become?) in the context of American, white-dominated society?" No "Sacred Cow" is speared in this almost Biblical, Job-like "confrontation" with real events and circumstances as experienced by this writer. Between these pages can be found real amelioration strategies for age-old "problems," particularly self-identity and taking back control over personal health and well-being.

4. Bircher-Benner, M. *Nutrition Plan for Raw Food and Juices*. Plainview, New York: Nash Publishing Co., 1972.

-Outline of the benefits of raw food diet by one of the pioneers in the field.

5. Bircher-Benner, M., *Eating Your Way to Health.* New York, New York: Viking-Penguin Books, 1961.

-Recipes and raw food philosophy along with background on Bircher-Benner Clinic.

6. Clark, Linda, *Know Your Nutrition.* New Canaan, CT 06940: Keats Publishing Co., 1973.

-Comprehensive nutrition course. Non-technical, very readable.

7. Davis, Adelle, *Let's Eat Right to Keep Fit.* Bergenfield, NJ 07621: New American Library, 1970.

-Davis's basic book on nutrition and natural health. Very informative. Includes tables of food composition.

8. Ibid.,, *You Can Get Well.* Simi, CA 93065; Lust Enterprises, Inc., 1975.

-A popular book on suggestions for eating for a variety of disease conditions. Also contains a food composition chart with foods, vitamins, minerals, and calories.

9. Diamond, Harvey and Marilyn, *Fit for Life.* New York, NY: Warner Books, Inc., 1985.

-Perhaps the most popular—and important—book of the 1980's. Credited with spawning the worldwide "wellness consciousness movement." Takes the wellness-conscious person, perhaps, 70% to 75% of the way to an optimum healthful living lifestyle. Mentored by T. C. Fry, the Diamonds cling closely to the basic precepts of Dr. Herbert M. Shelton and the Science of Natural Hygiene. Viewed by many as the best book available on the subject through 1985.

10. Doyle, Rodger and James Redding, *The Complete Food Handbook.* New York, NY 10003: Grove Press, 1976.

-Reference book containing 200 types of food, evaluated for nutritive value, processing effects, chemical additives, and environmental contaminants. Well organized and highly readable.

11. Elwood, Catherine, *Feel Like a Million.* New York, NY 10018: Simon & Schuster, 1956.

-Good beginning book on nutrition. The book is clearly written for understanding.

12. Fry, T. C., *The Great AIDS Hoax.* Austin, TX: Life Science Institute, 1989 (as revised).

-Important discussion on **"the nature and purpose of disease,"** such that serious questions are raised which, when answered, point to various other "causes of AIDS," rather than those promulgated in the media! Dr. Fry decries "the phony notion of 'contagion'" and "proves AIDS is unrelated to either sex or viruses." Important for long-term drug users and other substance abusers who are now attempting to cleanse their systems through fasting techniques. More importantly, perhaps, the book is hauntingly frank in sharing research that confirms, "If you are not aware of what is causing your problem, you are likely to never uncover a solution." The "message" is that medical research spending is, substantially, fraudulent.

13. Fulton, Dr. Alvenia Moody, founder and director of Fultonia Health and Fasting Institute, Chicago, *Fasting Made Simple*. Chicago, IL: Fultonia Press, 1979.

-A fundamental guide to a fasting regimen which states, in simplistic language, how to personally conduct a safe and therapeutic fast. Written by the guru of "wholistic (whole body/mind) health" who taught this author and Dick Gregory the art and science of therapeutic fasting.

14. Harris, Ben Charles, *Kitchen Medicines*. New York, NY 10018: Simon & Schuster.

-Extremely interesting and informative. Filled with surprises.

15. Hendler, M. D., Ph.D., and Sheldon, Saul, *The Complete Guide to Anti-Aging Nutrients*. New York, NY: Simon and Schuster, 1985.

-An excellent, rational look at the products and research of the "life extension movement." A realistic look at the claims for a variety of nutritional substances.

16. Hunter, Beatrice, *The Natural Foods Primer*. New York, NY: Simon and Schuster, 1972.

-A beginner's guide to raw foods. Includes preparation tips. Sufficiently descriptive to preclude taking a simplistic view.

17. Jensen, Bernard, D.C., N.D., *You Can Master Disease*. Solana Beach, CA: Bernard Jensen Publishing, 1976.

-Dr. Jensen has been in private practice since 1929 and has spent many years studying other cultures, lifestyles and eating habits. Through iridology he and his associates have developed "preventive therapeutics." Fundamental to the onset of disease conditions is diet. Dr. Jensen asserts: "Americans do not eat enough of the right kind of foods. One family in ten has a good diet, less than four in ten have passable diets, and more than fifty per cent have poor diets. The lack of the proper nutritional education program in grammar school, (junior high or middle school), high school and college is one of the contributing causes to this dilemma."

18. Kaslow, Arthur L., MD, *You Can Achieve Freedom From Chronic Disease*. California: J. P. Tarcher, Inc., 1979.

-A self-care program based on Dr. Kaslow's principles. Informative, very readable. Goes beyond nutrition, to form a truly wholistic program.

19. Katahn, Martin, Ph.D., *Beyond Diet*. London, New York, NY 10110: W. W. Norton & Company, 1984.

-No diet is the way to go. Avoid "low calorie" foods. These two statements sum up the focus of this book.

20. Kordel, Lelord, *Eat and Grow Younger*. New York, NY: World Publishing Company, 1962.

-Much ado is spent building a case for "powdered skim milk." Arguments in this volume should give the reader pause for thought.

21. Kugler, Hans, *Slowing Down the Aging Process*. New York, NY 10017: Pyramid Publications, 1975.

-Compilation of current studies and theories of aging. Section on diet and aging. Interesting and informative, but inconclusive perhaps.

22. Maelstrom, Stan D., N.D., M.T., *Own Your Own Body*. New Canaan, CT: Keats Publishing, Inc., 1977.

-"Your body belongs to you—not to your doctor, not to the sellers and advertisers of the food, drink and chemicals it takes in. Only you can make sure that your body reaches and stays at the peak of the vibrant good health that makes life truly worth living." Clearly, the author provides his own summary.

23. Passwater, Richard, *Supernutrition.* New York, NY 10018: Simon and Schuster, 1975.

-An informative book by a biochemist, on the relationship of dietary deficiency to disease. He recounts some interesting evidence regarding low cholesterol. However, Passwater misses an opportunity to comprehend the true correlation between diet and disease; like others before him, the paradigm just appears too simple.

24. Pearson, Durk and Shaw, Sandy, *Life Extension: A Practical Scientific Approach.* New York, NY: Warner Books, 1982.

-A virtual encyclopedia of the life extension movement. Packed with information. There are appropriate cautions and disclaimers added at the end of each chapter. Reader options remain clear throughout. In the *Companion* book that followed in 1984, two interesting original research studies added "fuel" to the life extension fire.

25. Rodale, J.J. & Staff, *Encyclopedia for Healthful Living*. Emmanus, PA 18049: Rodale Press, 1960.

-Discussion on a multitude of subject areas regarding diet and health by a pioneer in the area of natural health.

26. Scarborough, Dr. Robert L., Jr., *How to Feel Good and Stop the Aging Process.* Maryland: D.B.S. Publishers, 1981.

-Another informative program for achieving health and longevity. Includes exercise routines, perhaps a most critical consideration in any wellness effort.

27. Shelton, Herbert, N.D., *Food Combining Made Easy.* San Antonio, TX 78206: American Natural Hygiene Press, 1951.

-One of the leaders of the American Natural Hygiene movement summarizes his views of food combining. He includes a liberal amount of menus, which demonstrate the foci he describes. Easy to understand classification for foods, and detailed instructions on how to take your proteins, starch, and on eating fruits. Also discusses vegetables or "a salad a day." Dr. Shelton furthers distinguishes between 'right' and 'wrong' food combinations.

28. Ibid., *Vaccine and Serum Evils.* San Antonio, TX: Dr. Shelton's Health School, and Health Research (Mokelumne Hill, CA 95245), 1966.

-A very valuable book for mothers of small children, and for those traveling abroad, or those in service organizations who are "prevailed upon" to submit to the deadly practice of "a criminal operation…a filthy practice, born out of the ignorance and superstitions of the past and fathered by an ignorant impostor and fraud, palmed off on the world today as a scientific procedure." Obviously, Dr. Shelton disapproves of any injection/s, for whatever reason or justification that might be advanced under ill advice at best.

29. Ibid., *Fasting for the Renewal of Life.* Tampa, FL: American Natural Hygiene Society.

-Dr. Shelton gives scientific evidence how the body increases functions and eliminates symptoms in acute and chronic disease conditions. Also highly recommended for those concerned about "degenerative diseases."

30. Ibid., *The Science and Fine Art of Fasting*. San Antonio, TX: Willow Publishing, Inc., 1934 and Tampa, FL: American Natural Hygiene Society, 1978.

-Dr. Shelton explains the nature of disease, pointing out its relationship to toxicosis, and how the compilation of toxemia leads to so-called 'degenerative disease' conditions. He also provides guidance for those wishing to practice fasting as "a therapeutic way of life."

31. Ibid., *Getting Well.* Modelumne Hill, CA: Health Research and American Natural Hygiene Society (Tampa, FL).

-An earlier book by Dr. Herbert M. Shelton, but one of his 'classics' on the hygienic system of living in harmony with the laws of nature to effect the optimum results of a healthful lifestyle, free of disease and debilitation. Once 'the law of natural hygiene" is understood, Dr. Shelton makes clear the course for recovering from various 'disease conditions.'

32. Ibid., with Osward, Jean A., *Fasting for the Health of It.* Pueblo, CO: Nationwide Press, Ltd., 1983.

-Fascinating case studies of fasting and terrific results, from the March 1963 plane crash where two survivors lived for seven weeks just eating melted snow to the 58-year-old man who "had been taking thirty-five units of insulin daily for one year. On arrival his blood sugar level was 181. After his seven-day fast, his blood sugar dropped to 130 and he was able to control his sugar level without taking insulin."

33. Ibid., with Williard, Jo and Osward, Jean A., *Natural Hygiene Weight-Loss Diet Book.* New Canaan, CT: Keats Publishing, Inc., 1986.

-The dedication in this book is, perhaps, its most unique aspect: "To Herbert M. Shelton who revived and refined the philosophy and science of Natural Hygiene and who died on January 1, 1985, too soon to see this book in print."

34. Tilden, John H., MD, *Toxemia: The Basic Cause of Disease* (Abridged Edition). Tampa, FL: Natural Hygiene Press (A Division of American Natural Hygiene Society, Inc.), 1974.

-"In the process of tissue building—metabolism—there is cell building—anabolism—and cell destruction—catabolism. The broken down tissue is toxic and in health when nerve energy is normal, it is eliminated from the blood as fast as evolved. When nerve energy is dissipated from any cause, physical, mental or bad habits the body becomes enervated. When enervated, elimination is checked, causing a retention of toxins within the blood and tissues which we name toxemia." A man plucked out from among us—in a sense, like Jesus was—dedicated his life to teaching the simple true he had been inspired to teach, actually dying in process of preparing further teachings. Dr. Herbert M. Shelton is said to have died from "enervation," pressing to complete yet another book on Natural Hygiene, the science of healthful living in accord with Natural Law.

35. White, E. G., *Health and Happiness*. Los Angeles, CA 90048: Audio Visual Production (first published in 1905).

-A unique treatment juxtaposing "holistic health principles" with passages from the Bible. A very interesting book for those who wish to draw “a religious connection” to the recommended principles of good health.

Selected References

1. Afua, Queen, *Heal Thyself with Health and Longevity*. New York, NY: Helen Robinson/Heal Thyself, 1991.

2. Allen, Hannah, *Health and Rejuvenation*. Austin, TX: Life Science Soceity, 1975.

3. *Ibid., How to Keep Your Body Pure*. Austin, TX: Life Science Society, (unknown)

4. *Ibid., Toxemia Explained: The True Healing Art*. Life Science Society, (unknown)

5. *Ibid., The Great Water Controversy*. Life Science Society, (unknown)

6. *Ibid., Homemakers' Guide to Foods for Pleasure & Health and Handbook for Hygienic Living*. Chicago, IL 60613: Natural Hygiene Press, 1976.

7. Alexander, Peter, Editor, *William Shakespeare—The Complete Works*. London and Glasgow: Collins Clear-Type Press, 1965.

8. Alpert, Dr. Felicity, *The Gift of Life—A Manual for Living Longer*. Brisbane, Queensland (Australia): The Institute for the Advancement of Community Health PTY LTD, 1993.

9. Anderson, Greg, *50 Essential Things to Do When the Doctor Says It's Cancer*. New York, NY 10014: Penguin Books USA Inc., 1993.

10. Anderson, Henry L. N., *Helping Hand: Guide to Healthful Living*. Ikeja, Lagos: Anderson-Beverly Publishers, Ltd., 1992.

11. Ibid., *Organic Wellness Fasting Technique*. Beverly Hills, CA 90212-7219: BLI Publishers, 1992.

12. Ibid., *Revolutionary Urban Teaching*. Los Angeles, CA: American University Publishers, 1973.

13. Ibid., *Ihre Gesundheit liegt in Ihrer Hand*. D-2863 Ritterhude, West Germany: Waldthausen Verlag, 1992.

14. Ibid., *No Use Cryin'*. Los Angeles, CA 90015: Western Publishers, 1961.

15. Ibid., *Helping Hand: American Diet*. Tokyo: Tokai University Press, 1994.

16. Ibid., *Helping Hand: 8-Day Diets Programs for People Who Care About Wellness*. Pacific Palisades, CA: Publius Publishing, 1986.

17. *Ibid., African, Born in America*. Beverly Hills, CA 90212-7219: BLI Publishers, 1993. Introduction by Dick Gregory.

18. Baratan, R. K., Editor, *Trusteeship—The Indian Contribution to a New Social Order*. 600 014 Madras, India: Sriniketan (An Institution of National Education), 1979.

19. Baker, Arthur M., *Awakening Our Self-Healing Body—A Solution to the Health Care Crisis*. Los Angeles, CA 90035: Self Health Care Systems, 1994.

20. Baker, Dr. Elton and Elizabeth, M. A., *The Unmedical Book.* Saguache, CO 81149: Communication Creativity, 1987.

21. Berger, Stuart M., *How to Be Your Own Nutritionist.* New York, NY: Avon Books, 1987.

22. Blume, Harold S., *Are Waerland's Health Hand-Book.* CH-3000 Bern 6, Switzerland: Humata Publications, 1977.

23. Braude, Jacob M., *Braude's Treasury of Wit and Humor for All Occasions.* Paramus, NJ 07652: Prentice Hall, 1991.

24. Crick, Francis, *Life Itself—Its Origin and Nature.* London EC2A 2EN, England: Macdonald and Co. (Publishers) Ltd., 1982.

25. Chopra, Deepak, MD, *Ageless Body, Timeless Mind.* New York, NY: Harmony Books, 1993.

26. Davis, Adelle, *Let's Cook It Right.* New York, NY 10017: Harcourt Brace Jovanovich, Inc., 1970.

27. Ibid., *Let's Get Well.* New York, NY: Harcourt, Brace & World, Inc., 1965.

28. Diamond, Harvey and Marilyn, *Fit for Life.* New York, NY: Warner Books, Inc., 1985.

29. Ibid., *Fit for Life II: Living Health.* New York, NY: Warner Books, Inc., 1987.

30. Ibid., *Fit for Life: A New Way of Eating*

31. Diamond, Harvey, *You Can Prevent Breast Cancer!* San Diego, CA 92122: ProMotion Publishing, 1995.

32. Diamond, John, MD, *Your Body Doesn't Lie.* New York, NY 10019: Warner Books, 1980.

33. Ellison, F. Fern, *Your Health and Wealth Is Your Business.* San Diego, CA 92129: Brenner Information Group, 1989.

34. Fox, Arnold, MD, *The Beverly Hills Medical Diet.* St. Louis Park, MN 55426: Chain-Pinkham Books, 1981.

35. Fox, Arnold, MD and Fox, Barry, *Wake Up! You're Alive.* Deerfield Beach, FL 33442: Health Communications, Inc., 1988.

36. Fredericks, Carlton, Ph.D. and Bailey, Herbert, *Food Facts and Fallacies.* New York, NY 10003: Arco Publishing Company, Inc., 1978.

37. Fry, T. C., *Program for Dynamic Health.* Chicago, IL: Natural Hygiene Press, 1974.

38. Ibid., *The Great AIDS Hoax.* Austin, TX: Life Science Institute, 1987 (Rev. 1989)

39. Ibid., with Shelton, Dr. Herbert M., and Others, *Reversing Arthritis.* Manchaca, TX 78652-0609: Health Excellence, 1992.

40. Fulton, Alvenia M., ND, Ph.D., *The Fasting Primer*. Chicago, IL 60602: B.C.A. Publishing Corp., 1978.

41. Ibid., *Vegetarianism: Fact or Myth? Eating to Live*. Chicago, IL 60602: B.C.A. Publishing Corp., 1978.

42. Goss, Dr. Paul, *Forever Young*. Compton, CA: New Body Publishers, 1985.

43. Goston, Empress Verdiacee "Tiari," *Return of the Ancient Ones*. C/o P.O. Box 4277, Inglewood: via U.S.A. Postal Code 90309-4277: Washitaw Publishing Company, 1993.

44. Huang, Wayne H., Translator, *The Diamond Sutra*. Hacienda Heights, CA 92745: CUBT Publishing, 1993.

45. Jensen, Bernard, Ph.D., *Vibrant Health from Your Kitchen*. Escondido, CA 92025: Bernard Jensen, Publisher, 1986.

46. Ibid., *Doctor-Patient Handbook*. Escondido, CA 92027: Bernard Jensen Enterprises, 1984.

47. Ibid., *Tissue Cleansing Through Bowel Management*: Escondido, CA 90225: Jensen Publishing, 1980.

48. Karpinski, Gloria D., *Where Two Worlds Touch*. New York, NY: Random House/Ballentine Books, 1990.

49. King, Coretta Scott, *The Words of Martin Luther King, Jr.* New York, NY 10017: Newmarket Press, 1983.

50. Kordel, Lelord, *Eat and Grow Younger.* New York, NY 10016: Manor Books, Inc., 1962.

51. Krimm, Irwinn F., Ps.D., *Health, Success and Happiness for You.* Los Angeles, CA 90015: Western Publishers, Ltd., 1963.

52. Lyman, Howard F., *Mad Cowboy.* New York, NY 10020: Scribner (Simon and Schuster Inc.), 1998.

53. Nahm, Andrew C., Ph.D., *A Panorama of 5000 Years: Korean History.* Elizabeth, NJ 07208 (USA)/Seoul, Korea 725-7554: Hollym Corporation, Publishers, 1983.

54. Null, Gary and Staff, *Food Combining Handbook.* Denver, CO 80217: The Berkley Publishing Group (NY 10016), 1983.

55. Osterlund, David (Introduction by), *The Constitution of the United States of America.* New York, NY: Barnes and Noble, 1995.

56. Owen, Bob L., Ph.D., *The Pure Cure for Arthritis.* Cannon Beach, OR 97110: Health Digest Books, 1997.

57. Ibid., *Roger's Recovery from AIDS.* Malibu, CA 90265: Davar Publishers, 1987.

58. Pauling, Linus, *Vitamin C, The Common Cold and The Flu.* New York, NY 10016: Berkley Publishing Corporation, 1981.

59. Pierce, Carson E., *What I Would Do If I Had Cancer Again.* Los Angeles, CA: Carlson E. Pierce Organization, 1992.

60. Ponder, Catherine, *The Dynamic Laws of Healing.* Marina del Rey, CA 90294: DeVORSS and Company, 1966.

61. Rader, William, MD, *No-Diet Program for Permanent Weight Loss.* New York, NY 10019: Warner Communications Company, 1981.

62. "*Reappraising AIDS,*" The Group for the Scientific Reappraisal of the AIDS/HIV Hypothesis: La Jolla, CA 92037, 1997.

63. Robins, John, *Reclaiming Our Health.* Tiburon, CA 94920: H. J. Kramer, Inc., 1996.

64. Sale, George, *The Koran of Mohammed.* Chicago, IL: Regan Publishing Corporation, (year unknown).

65. Shelton, Herbert M., *The Science and Fine Art of Fasting.* Bridgeport, CT 06604: Natural Hygiene Press, 1978 (5th Revised Edition).

66. Ibid., *Syphilis—Werewolf of Medicine.* Mokelumne Hill, CA 95245: Health Research Publication, (year unidentifiable).

67. Ibid., *Vaccine and Serum Evils.* Mokelumne Hill, CA 95245: Dr. Shelton's Health School/Health Research, 1966.

68. Ibid., *The Original Natural Hygiene Weight Loss Diet Book.* New Canaan, CT 06840: Keats Publishing, Inc. 1986.

69. Ibid., *Getting Well.* Mokelumne Hill, CA: Health Research, (date unknown).

70. Ibid., *Human Life, Its Philosophy and Laws.* Mokehumne Hill, CA 95245: Health Research, 1928, 1942.

71. Ibid., *Superior Nutrition.* San Antonio, TX: Willow Publishing, Inc., 1982.

72. Ibid., *Fasting: Fastest Way to Super Health and Rejuvenation.* Austin, TX: Life Science Society, 1975.

73. Ibid., *The Science and Fine Art of Good Nutrition*, Vol. II. Oldsmar, FL 33557: Natural Hygiene Press, 1984.

74. Snodgrass, Beth, *Overcoming Asthma.* Manchaca, TX 78652-0609: Health Excellence Systems, (unknown).

75. Starr, Amber (and Loomis, Evarts, MD), *The Meadowlark Cookbook II.* Hemet, CA 92343: Friendly Hills Fellowship Press, (after) 1959.

76. Strassberg, Peter M., MD, *The 100-Year Diet.* Great Neck, NY 11021: Todd and Honeywell, Inc., 1985.

77. Stillman, Irwin Maxwell and Baker, Samon Sinclair, *The Doctor's Quick INCHES-OFF DIET.* New York, NY 10017: Dell Publishing Co., Inc., 1970.

78. Ibid., *The Doctor's Quick Weight Loss Diet.* New York, NY: Dell, 1971.

79. Tilden, John H., MD, *Toxemia: The Basic Cause of Disease.* Chicago, IL 60613: American Natural Hygiene Society, Inc., 1974.

80. Thomas, Richard, *The Essiac Report.* Los Angeles, CA 90069: The Alternative Treatment Information Network, 1993.

81. Verdiacee, Empress, *Return of the Ancient Ones.* Washitaw Publishing Company: P.O. Box 4277, Inglewood, CA 90309-4277, 1993 ($50.00 post paid).

82. Wade, Carlson, *Miracle Protein: Secret of Natural Cell-Tissue Rejuvenation.* West Nyack, NY: Parker Publishing Company, Inc., 1975.

83. White, E. G., *Health and Happiness.* Jemison, AL 35085: Audio Visual Production (IBE Retail Marketing Services), 1984.

84. Whitehouse, Dr. Geoffrey T., *Stop Poisoning Yourself!* London SW7, England: Universal-Tandem Publishing Company Limited, 1968.

85. Yogi, His Holiness Maharishi Mahesh, *Maharishi Forum of Natural Law and National Law for DOCTORS.* India: Age of Enlightenment Publications, 1995.

86. Zilkha, Dr. J. G., *Management of Self-Health and Fitness*. South Church, Durham: The Pentland Press Ltd., 1993.

Index

About the Author

Henry L. N. Anderson is the author of ten published books and a half dozen unpublished manuscripts. In 1962 he registered with the Screen Writers Guild, Hollywood, CA, a 39-episode treatment entitled, "The Solomons," a Negro-family sitcom for the post-Amos 'N Andy era, which he believes was the basis of what the public came to know as "The Jeffersons." Anderson has never been compensated for his pioneering work.

He began writing as a teenager and won his first literary award while in high school for a poem entitled, "On Sunday Morn," selected and published in the *Intercollegian*, magazine of the campus YMCA movement. His first novel, *No Use Cryin'*, was first published in 1961; a second novel, *World War III*, underwent a title change to *When They Turn to Loving* and remains unpublished. Also, yet unpublished is a 50-year collection of poems titled *Mood Poetry for Everyone*, reminiscent of Shakespeare down to modern "rap" lyrics.

Henry L. N. Anderson is an educator, having taught school at all levels; and for the past 30 years has been in university administration, as department chair, academic vice president, president, and as university chancellor. His travels have taken him around the world several times; and he has lectured on "wellness issues" in several countries. He produced and hosted the award-winning television show, "Organic Wellness Crusade" (1991), and is the creator, writer, director, producer, executive producer, and host of a one-hour television interview show entitled "Wellness Issues."

Dr. Anderson's public service includes (transitional) Emperial Administrator and Minister of Education of ***Uaxashaktun (Empire Washitaw) de Dugdahmoundyah*** Nation; and he headed the Washitaw Nation's delegation to the "Indigenous Peoples Conference" at Geneva, Switzerland, July 24-27, 2001 and delivered a formal speech.

In his private life, he is the father of three grown children, and the grandfather of eight. He lives in Los Angeles with his wife, Dr. Margie N. Johnson.

About the Book

"The Nature of Disease is 'the last word' I will make on the subject of disease, because I have taken the pretense out and striped away the 'mystery.' What the peoples of the world consume determines what happens to them, health-wise. 'Disease' is no more or no less than the consequences of internal poisoning, **believe it or not**! And, as T.C. Fry so aptly put it: 'Disease would not occur so long as its causes are not engaged.'"
–The Author

I believe I have finally come across a book that lays out the truth, whether I adapt it to my personal lifestyle or not. At least, I feel I now can know what the truth is!"

—Rev. Dr. Frank C. Maddox, African Methodist Episcopal Church, Marion, S.C.

"I know what the book is saying; and I clearly understand my options. I also believe anyone reading the book will also understand the options. I have tried the methodology and I was empowered." —Ileana A. Woods, North Hollywood, CA

"Young people who are now programmed to care so little for their precious physical bodies need to discover this book right now, before their brains, livers, kidneys, digestive systems and all their other vital organs have been damaged and partly destroyed by medication, hard drugs, and nutrition-less food...."
—V. V. Vetrano, MD, Barksdale, TX

"Perhaps as important an illustration to the wisdom of Dr. Anderson's book lies in its implied refutation of the 'contagion theory.' 'Viral attack' is a concocted myth. First, virii are dead and therefore inert. These genomic materials are derived from mitochondria that expired with the death of the cell of which they were a part. Genomes called virii (viruses) are the remains of the onslaught of the cells' disintegrative lysosomes released simultaneous to cellular death. Dead materials attack nothing! In the case of so-called cytomegalovirus, everything is the same except that the origin of a giant genome was the cell nucleus itself."

–T. C. Fry, Wellsboro, PA, 1995

"I had many questions about Dr. Anderson's book; but, the more I read the fewer questions remained. Now, a lot of what I always thought is making more sense; and, I am empowered to design my own 'disease-prevention' program.

–Georgia Washington, Los Angeles County, CA

American University Publishers
P.O. Box 4277
Inglewood, CA 90309-4277

Call (310) 671-0634 to order

NAME____

ADDRESS____

CITY____

STATE__________________ZIP________________________

(Please add shipping charges of $5 first book and $1.00 ea. additional)

Total Amount Enclosed $.................

................check

................credit card...............Visa...........Master Card

Card Number...

Name on Card..

Expiration Date...